MW00904223

Neonatal Intensive Care Nursing Exam Study Guide

RNC-NIC Review Book for the Neonatal Intensive Care Nursing Exam

Emma Hayes
© 2023-2024
Printed in USA.

Disclaimer:

Content

Why do you need to be RNC-NIC Certified?

Being RNC-NIC (Registered Nurse Certified in Neonatal Intensive Care) certified is essential for several reasons.

- Firstly, it signifies that a nurse has completed the required education and training in neonatal intensive care nursing, ensuring their competence in providing specialized care to critically ill newborns.

- This certification also demonstrates the nurse's commitment to maintaining the highest standards of patient care and professional development in this specific field.

- Moreover, employers often prioritize hiring RNC-NIC certified nurses, as it assures them of the nurse's expertise and ability to effectively manage complex neonatal conditions.

- Overall, being RNC-NIC certified enhances job prospects, professional credibility, and ultimately leads to the delivery of safe and specialized care to neonates.

<u>Willing To Join Our Author Panel?</u>

Dear Registered Nurses,

We would like to invite you to join our 'Panel Of Authors'.

First of all, Thank you for your hard work and dedication to your patients. We know that the hours are long and the workload is demanding, but you do it with grace and dignity. Your compassion is evident in the way you treat your patients, and we are grateful for all that you do.

We believe that your expertise and experience as nurses will be a valuable contribution to our books. Our goal is to provide valuable content that helps nurses to step forward in their career development. This is a unique opportunity to share your expertise with other nurses and help shape the future of nursing.

The requirements for joining our panel of authors are as follows:
- A minimum experience of 8 years in nursing
- Proper certification from a renowned organization
- Good writing and teaching skills
- Enthusiasm in sharing knowledge

If you meet these requirements and are interested in joining our panel, please send us your resume along with a writing sample for our review to propublisher@zohomail.com . We would be happy to have you on board!

We are happy that our panel of authors can provide the best content because they are experienced and passionate about nursing. We would love for you to join our panel of authors and help us continue to provide quality content for nurses. You will also be able to connect with other nurses from around the world and build a network of support. Undoubtedly, this will be a great opportunity for you to make a difference in the nursing profession.

Thank You.

Why is this book the right choice for you to clear the RNC-NIC Exam?

Latest Study Guide:
If you are looking for an up-to-date study guide for the RNC-NIC Exam, then look no further than this book. This book provides everything you need to know to ace the exam with tons of practice questions to help you prepare. This book is also constantly updated to ensure that it always covers the latest information on the exam as per the outline provided by the NCC ®.

RNC-NIC® TEST CONTENT OUTLINE

1. General Assessment (9%) Maternal Risk Factors and Birth History Physical and Gestational Age Assessment

2. General Management (44%) Resuscitation and Stabilization Fluids and Electrolytes and Glucose Homeostasis Nutrition and Feeding Oxygenation, Ventilation and Acid Base Homeostasis Thermoregulation and Integumentary Pharmacology, Pharmacokinetics and Pharmacodynamics Neuroprotective and Neurodevelopmental Care Infection and Immunology

3. Assess & Manage Pathophysiologic States (39%) Cardiovascular Respiratory Gastrointestinal and Gastrourinate Hematopoietic Neurological/Neuromuscular Genetic, Metabolic and Endocrine Head, Eye, Ear, Nose Throat

4. Psychosocial Support (5%) Discharge Management, Family Centered Care, Grieving, Palliative Care, Mental Health

5. Professional Issues (3%) including: Evidence Based Practice, Legal/Ethical, Patient Safety, Quality Improvement

Experienced Set of Authors:
There are many reasons to choose this book over others, but one of the most important is that it is written by experienced authors who are RNC-NIC Certified. The authors of this book have a wealth of experience in taking and passing exams, and we have used our knowledge to create a study guide that is comprehensive and easy to follow.
With our experienced authors and comprehensive coverage, our book is the best way to prepare for this important test.

Detailed rationale for the answer:
We provide an in-depth explanation for each question, so you can understand not only the correct answer but also why it is correct. This book also gives you an ample amount of practice to help you feel confident on exam day.

Similar Question Format as that in the actual exam:

One of the most important features of this book is that the questions and answers follow the same pattern as the actual exam. This is extremely important because you need to be familiar with the format of the exam to do well on it.

Fine Tunes your thinking:
Going through the questions, answers and explanations repeatedly will sharpen your thinking and understanding ability. This will help you to understand the root of the question in the RNC-NIC Exam and make the right selection of the answer.

Clear and Concise:
This RNC-NIC Prep is written in simple language and is not overly technical. This sets this book apart from other study materials because when you are studying for the RNC-NIC Exam, you need to be able to understand the material without getting bogged down in details. This book will help you do just that. This combination of easy-to-understand language and practical testing will help you be successful on the RNC-NIC exam.

Magical Steps to Pass the RNC-NIC Exam with Ease:

1. Belief: You must believe that you can pass the RNC-NIC exam with ease. This belief will help you stay focused and motivated throughout your studies. We help build your confidence by giving you the feel of attending virtual exams in our book, making you familiar with the type of questions that will be asked in the exam, and giving you a thorough idea about all the topics as specified by NCC®.

2. Visualization: Visualize yourself passing the RNC-NIC exam with flying colors. This will help you stay positive and focused on your goal. Taking multiple tests and solving various questions will help improve your positivity and confidence. We try our best to improve your positivity.

3. Study: Make sure to study all the material thoroughly. Quality Learning is more important than Quantity Learning. Time yourself when you take tests and try to complete them within the stipulated time.

4. Practice: The more you practice the more is the chance of passing the exam. By doing this, you will get a feel for the types of questions that will be asked and how to best answer them. We have an abundant number of questions for you to practice.

5. Relax: On the day of the exam, make sure to relax and stay calm. This will help you think more clearly and perform at your best.

Smart Learning with Trust in Yourself will make Success knock at your door! All the Best!

Neonatal Intensive Care Nursing Exam Practice Questions

Question 1: A newborn baby, immediately after birth, shows signs of severe blueness due to decreased blood flow to the lungs and a mixture of oxygen-rich and oxygen-poor blood. The baby also has difficulty feeding or crying, which further intensifies the blueness. What condition do these symptoms suggest?

A) Atrial Septal Defect

B) Ventricular Septal Defect

C) Tetralogy of Fallot

Question 2: How would you describe the characteristics of gestational hypertension?

A) Hypertension after 20 weeks with proteinuria

B) Hypertension before 20 weeks with proteinuria

C) Hypertension after 20 weeks without proteinuria

Question 3: "What method can be utilized to evaluate the autonomic function in a newborn baby?"

A) Blood pressure monitoring

B) Heart rate variability

C) Body temperature measurement

Question 4: What heart disorder could lead to weak pulses in the extremities and a decrease in the temperature of the limbs?

A) Ventricular Septal Defect

B) Tetralogy of Fallot

C) Hypoplastic left heart syndrome (HLHS)

Question 5: What is the standard arterial blood gas (ABG) measurement for PaO2 in a newborn baby?

A) 60 to 80 mmHg

B) 80 to 100 mmHg

C) 40 to 60 mmHg

Question 6: What would be considered a hyperglycemic condition in a premature newborn in terms of blood glucose level?

A) <100 mg/dL

B) 100-120 mg/dL

C) >150 mg/dL

Question 7: What does a positive result on a Kleihauer-Betke test suggest, especially after a mother has experienced a traumatic event like a car accident?

A) Reduced chance of fetal distress

B) Decreased risk of maternal infection

C) Elevated likelihood of premature delivery

Question 8: "What contributes the most to the level of noise in a Neonatal Intensive Care Unit (NICU)?"

A) The sound of medical equipment

B) Conversation

C) The crying of babies

Question 9: "If the parents of a newborn baby boy, let's call him Ethan, have decided against circumcision, what advice should be incorporated into their care guidelines?"

A) The foreskin should not be touched or cleaned at all.

B) The foreskin should be completely retracted for cleaning and the area should be dried well.

C) The foreskin should be partially retracted for cleaning and the area should be left moist.

Question 10: What combination of medications can be safely administered together via an intravenous route?

A) Phenytoin (Dilantin) with Lactated Ringer's solution

B) Phenytoin (Dilantin) with Normal Saline

C) Phenytoin (Dilantin) with D5W

Question 11: "What is an instance of the didactic caregiving pattern?"

A) Ignoring the infant's cues

B) Stimulating the infant

C) Overfeeding the infant

Question 12: "Which patient situation does NOT require the use of mechanical ventilation?"

A) 28-week infant weighing 1200 g, respiratory rate 60/min, grunting, and flaring

B) Infant at 34 weeks, with a weight of 2400 g, having a respiratory rate of 42/min, placed in an oxyhood on 30% FiO2.

C) Full-term infant with meconium aspiration syndrome, respiratory rate 70/min, cyanotic

Question 13: When administering IV ganciclovir to a newborn diagnosed with congenital cytomegalovirus infection, what is the recommended duration for the infusion?

A) 90 minutes

B) 30 minutes

C) 60 minutes

Question 14: What condition would likely occur if a near-term fetus, let's call him Baby Anthony, generates between 200 to 400 mL of urine each day?

A) Oligohydramnios

B) Hydrops fetalis

C) Polyhydramnios

Question 15: During labor, at what rate would a fetal heart be categorized as experiencing tachycardia?

A) >160 bpm for ≥10 minutes

B) <120 bpm for ≥10 minutes

C) 120-160 bpm for ≥10 minutes

Question 16: "What is the approximate distance at which a full-term newborn's eyes can focus?"

A) 25 to 30 inches

B) 15 to 20 inches

C) 8 to 10 inches

Question 17: If a neonate is born prematurely, at what gestational age is it necessary to shield their eyes from light?

A) 32 weeks of gestation

B) 36 weeks of gestation

C) 28 weeks of gestation

Question 18: In the case of a newborn baby whose mother is infected with hepatitis B, what is the recommended timeframe for the infant to receive both the hepatitis B immune globulin and the hepatitis B vaccine to prevent transmission of the disease?

A) 24 hours

B) 12 hours

C) 48 hours

Question 19: "Which among the listed congenital heart anomalies is recognized as a condition causing cyanosis?"

A) Ventricular Septal Defect

B) Tetralogy of Fallot

C) Atrial Septal Defect

Question 20: "What medical condition would prevent the use of nasal Continuous Positive Airway Pressure (CPAP)?"

A) Bronchopulmonary dysplasia

B) Choanal atresia

C) Respiratory distress syndrome

Question 21: "What is the potential outcome for infants in the Neonatal Intensive Care Unit (NICU) when a cycled lighting system (bright in the daytime and dim at night) is implemented?"

A) Infants having longer periods of sleep deprivation

B) Infants being able to feed sooner

C) Infants experiencing higher levels of stress

Question 22: When will a child, who has been diagnosed with late congenital syphilis, typically start to exhibit symptoms?

A) During the first year of life

B) Post the second year of existence

C) Immediately after birth

Question 23: What is the caloric content per deciliter of colostrum?

A) 45

B) 85

C) 67

Question 24: What is the noise level recommended by the AAP for a Neonatal Intensive Care Unit (NICU)?

A) <60 dB

B) <30 dB

C) <45 dB

Question 25: What type of examination should the parents or caregivers of a newborn, who has been treated for bacterial meningitis, be advised to arrange for their baby within a timeframe of 4 to 6 weeks after discharge?

A) Hearing test

B) Skin sensitivity test

C) Vision test

Question 26: "What is one of the impacts of using cycled light in the Neonatal Intensive Care Unit?"

A) Decreased heart rate

B) Enhanced visual acuity

C) Increased risk of infection

Question 27: Can you explain how an omphalocele differs from a gastroschisis?

A) An omphalocele refers to the protrusion of abdominal contents through the umbilicus, while in a gastroschisis, the abdominal organs lack a protective membrane covering

B) A gastroschisis occurs when the abdominal contents protrude through the umbilicus, but an omphalocele occurs when there is a membrane covering the abdominal organs.

C) Both omphalocele and gastroschisis are conditions where the abdominal contents protrude through the umbilicus and are covered by a membrane.

Question 28: What medical condition is a newborn, who is significantly larger than the average size for his gestational age, more likely to be susceptible to?

A) Congenital heart disease

B) Asthma

C) Shoulder dystocia

Question 29: "What is the primary reason for sudden kidney damage in newborns?"

A) Overhydration

B) Perinatal asphyxia

C) Genetic disorders

Question 30: What is the typical physiological reaction when a premature baby, born at 34 weeks of gestation, experiences hyperthermia?

A) Decreased heart rate

B) Vasoconstriction

C) Vasodilation

Question 31: "What is the initial diagnostic test that should be conducted when a newborn baby, for instance, baby Daniel, experiences a seizure?"

A) Conduct a hearing test

B) Blood glucose

C) Perform a skin biopsy

Question 32: What are the established advantages of the kangaroo care method, excluding 'More rapid PDA closure'?

A) Reduced maternal-infant bonding

B) Accelerated PDA closure

C) Increased risk of infection

Question 33: A week following his birth, a newborn baby, whom we'll call Ethan, presents with a state of near-unconsciousness, protruding anterior fontanel, seizures, and impairments in his cranial nerves. What could these symptoms indicate?

A) Neonatal jaundice

B) Congenital heart disease

C) Late-onset meningitis

Question 34: What is a potential risk factor for the onset of severe enterovirus disease?

A) Age above 2 years old

B) High platelet count

C) Hemoglobin less than 0.7 g/dL

Question 35: For a full-term baby who is breastfed, such as baby Emma, how much of the total feeding can be achieved from each breast within the initial 5 minutes of active nursing by the time she reaches 3 months old?

A) 80% to 90%

B) 100% to 110%

C) 50% to 60%

Question 36: What does it entail to be a conscientious and accountable neonatal intensive care nurse?

A) Focusing only on the physical well-being of the newborn

B) Maintaining up-to-date knowledge and skills

C) Ignoring parental concerns and focusing solely on medical procedures

Question 37: In line with the guidelines set by the American Academy of Pediatrics (AAP), it is suggested that all newborns weighing _____ undergo eye examinations to identify any indications of retinopathy of prematurity.?

A) All newborns regardless of weight

B) Newborns weighing ≤1,500 g

C) Newborns weighing ≥2,500 g

Question 38: In what circumstances would it be appropriate to administer surfactant to a newborn?

A) To infants who are sleeping excessively

B) To infants in severe respiratory distress that did not respond to CPAP

C) To infants who have a mild cold

Question 39: What is the typical age by which a newborn diagnosed with autosomal-recessive polycystic kidney disease is expected to progress to end-stage renal disease?

A) Early to mid-childhood

B) Within the first year of life

C) Late adolescence or early adulthood

Question 40: A baby boy, newly born, has been identified with a condition called neonatal testicular torsion, resulting in the loss of one testicle. The other testicle remains unaffected. The parents, concerned about their son's future fertility, are seeking advice. What would be the most suitable response to their query?

A) There is a very high chance of this causing fertility issues long-term.

B) The loss of one testicle will definitely result in infertility.

C) The potential for long-term fertility implications due to this is considerably minimal.

Question 41: When do the signs of transient tachypnea of the newborn (TTN) typically start to show?

A) 72 hours

B) Immediately after birth

C) 36 hours

Question 42: In the event of a car accident, a pregnant woman, let's call her Lisa, suffers from abruptio placenta. What condition should Lisa be closely observed for as a result of this?

A) Gestational diabetes

B) Postpartum coagulopathy and hemorrhage

C) Hypertensive disorders of pregnancy

Question 43: If a preterm newborn, let's call him Baby Michael, is receiving total parenteral nutrition and an extra 2 g/kg/day of protein is included in his basic intake, how many more nonprotein energy kilocalories will be necessary?

A) 30

B) 10

C) 20

Question 44: What is the implication of a high serum lactate level in a baby being cared for in the Neonatal Intensive Care Unit?

A) Increased risk of hyperactivity

B) Lowered risk of infection

C) Heightened Mortality Risk

Question 45: During the mid-20th century, specifically the 1940s and 1950s, can you identify the primary reason for childhood blindness in the United States?

A) Genetic disorders

B) Retinopathy of prematurity (ROP)

C) Vitamin A deficiency

Question 46: What would be a sign of Hirschsprung disease in a newborn baby?

A) Excessive weight gain in the first week

B) Frequent and uncontrollable crying episodes

C) Failure to pass meconium in 48 hours

Question 47: "What is the crucial step to remember when changing the diaper of a newborn baby diagnosed with osteogenesis imperfecta?"

A) Lift by the buttocks

B) Lift the baby by the legs

C) Lift the baby by the arms

Question 48: In a scenario where a newborn baby, let's call him baby Noah, requires a medication dosage of 40 mg/kg/day, split into two doses, and baby Noah's weight is 2.5 kg, how much medication would each dose contain?

A) 60 mg

B) 50 mg

C) 70 mg

Question 49: What is the appropriate ratio of cuff width to arm circumference when utilizing an oscillometric device to track a neonate's blood pressure?

A) 0.5 (1:2)

B) 1.0 (1:1)

C) 0.75 (3:4)

Question 50: What type of heat loss might occur if a newborn, for instance baby Mia, is laid down on a chilly surface?

A) Radiative

B) Evaporative

C) Conductive

Question 51: Under what circumstances should a surfactant be given to a newborn?

A) To infants who are suffering from mild dehydration

B) To infants who have a common cold

C) To neonates in severe respiratory distress unresponsive to CPAP

Question 52: For a newborn baby with an extremely low birth weight (ELBW), when does the passage of meconium typically take place?

A) Within the first 24 hours of birth

B) Birth to 5 days postpartum

C) After one week of birth

Question 53: "What substance is typically utilized in diagnosing a newborn with a congenital cytomegalovirus infection?"

A) Urine

B) Saliva

C) Cerebrospinal Fluid

Question 54: "For a newborn baby experiencing respiratory distress, when is the optimal period to administer surfactant?"

A) Immediately after the baby starts crying

B) Within 1 hour of birth

C) After 24 hours of birth

Question 55: At what stage of gestation does a baby typically develop the ability to coordinate sucking and swallowing?

A) 40 to 42 weeks of gestation

B) 33 to 36 weeks of gestation

C) 20 to 24 weeks of gestation

Question 56: What set of symptoms typically characterizes the maternal condition known as HELLP syndrome?

A) Frequent urination, excessive thirst, unexplained weight loss

B) Breakdown of red blood cells, increased hepatic enzyme levels, and a reduction in platelets

C) High blood pressure, excessive weight gain, protein in the urine

Question 57: What does a lactic acid level of 40 mg/dL (4.44 mmol/L) suggest in a newborn baby, named Lily, who is suffering from congestive heart failure?

A) Hyperglycemia

B) Hypoperfusion

C) Hypercalcemia

Question 58: What is the recommended timeframe for conducting a screening test for phenylketonuria (PKU)?

A) 24 to 72 hours

B) Immediately after birth

C) 1 to 2 weeks after birth

A) 1 day

B) 7 days

C) 14 days

Question 59: **"What is typically the primary reason for direct hyperbilirubinemia in a newborn baby?"**

A) Exposure to cold temperatures

B) Liver immaturity

C) Inadequate breast milk intake

Question 60: **Which option correctly indicates the suitable daily calorie intake for the corresponding baby?**

A) Healthy infant weighing 2500 g, fed 55 cc of expressed human milk via gavage every three hours.

B) Healthy 2500 g infant receiving 65 cc expressed human milk by gavage every 2 hours

C) Healthy 2500 g infant receiving 45 cc expressed human milk by gavage every 4 hours

Question 61: **"In newborn babies like little Emma, where is the primary site for the biotransformation or metabolism of medications?"**

A) Heart

B) Liver

C) Kidneys

Question 62: **Why would a preterm newborn, suffering from high blood sugar levels, be administered infusions of amino acids?**

A) To stimulate newborn's secretion of insulin

B) To increase the newborn's body weight

C) To enhance the newborn's immune system

Question 63: **In a newborn baby diagnosed with neonatal abstinence syndrome, who is experiencing acute withdrawal from alcohol, within what time period should we expect to see the onset of signs and symptoms?**

A) 24-48 hours after birth

B) 3-12 hours after birth

C) 1-2 weeks after birth

Question 64: **'What is the primary objective of allowing controlled hypercapnia in the prevention of bronchopulmonary dysplasia or chronic lung disease in neonates?**

A) To stimulate the production of red blood cells in neonates

B) To increase the blood pressure in neonates

C) To circumvent the need for intubation and ventilation or to allow for a reduced tidal volume.

Question 65: **When should a central line be suggested for the delivery of total parenteral nutrition (TPN), considering the duration of TPN is extended?**

Question 66: **"What is the suggested method when performing endotracheal suctioning on a newborn baby?"**

A) Ventilate the neonate before performing any suction event.

B) Perform a single suction event before ventilating the neonate.

C) Perform multiple suction events before ventilating the neonate.

Question 67: **"What is NOT considered a possible hazard when utilizing an extracorporeal membrane oxygenation (ECMO) device?"**

A) Electrolyte imbalance

B) Infection from the ECMO circuit

C) Hemorrhage from cannulation sites

Question 68: **What are the cut off values on the World Health Organization (WHO) growth chart that signify abnormal growth?**

A) 10th and 90th percentiles

B) 2nd and 98th percentiles

C) 5th and 95th percentiles

Question 69: **What would suggest that a newborn baby, let's say baby Anthony, has an inguinal hernia instead of a hydrocele if he has a scrotal mass?**

A) The mass is only visible when the baby cries or strains

B) The mass disappears when the baby is calm and relaxed

C) The mass can be diminished through applied pressure.

Question 70: **In a full-term newborn, what is the usual count of stratum corneum layers found in their epidermis?**

A) 50 to 60

B) 30 to 40

C) 10 to 20

Question 71: **Which method is most effective for conducting a screening for critical congenital heart disease?**

A) Pulse Oximeter

B) Auscultation with a stethoscope

C) Blood pressure monitor

Question 72: **'What is considered a standard rating on the fetal biophysical profile?'**

A) Three or more separate fetal movements in 30 minutes

B) Five or more separate fetal movements in 10 minutes

C) Two or less separate fetal movements in 30 minutes

Question 73: What is the recommended course of action for a newborn if the amniotic fluid is found to be stained with meconium at the time of delivery?

A) Standard neonatal resuscitation procedures

B) Administration of antibiotics immediately

C) Immediate intubation and mechanical ventilation

Question 74: What is the most effective method for diagnosing an early-onset group B streptococcal infection in a newborn?

A) Blood or cerebrospinal fluid culture

B) X-ray imaging

C) Urine test

Question 75: A neonate, born prematurely at 30 weeks, is about to be taken off the ventilator and shifted to nasal high-flow oxygen therapy. If the baby's weight is 1.4 kg, what should be the initial flow rate for the oxygen therapy?

A) 2 L/min

B) 3 L/min

C) 4 L/min

Question 76: In the context of performing bedside glucose tests to evaluate low blood sugar levels, what should the point-of-care glucose value be multiplied by to estimate the plasma glucose level?

A) 1.25

B) 0.89

C) 1.11

Question 77: The parents of a newborn baby are inquiring about PKU and its importance in the newborn screening process. What would be the most appropriate explanation to provide them?

A) PKU is a minor condition that doesn't require immediate attention.

B) PKU is a routine test that is not of much importance in the newborn screening process.

C)PKU is a potentially life-threatening condition, hence its screening is strongly advised.

Question 78: What is the standard head circumference for a newborn baby?

A) 40 to 45 cm

B) 20 to 25 cm

C) 32 to 38 cm

Question 79: "For which group of newborns does the American Academy of Pediatrics suggest the administration of Vitamin K shots?"

A) Only for neonates born to mothers with a history of drug use

B) All neonates

C) Only for neonates with a birth weight of less than 2.5 kg

Question 80: A newborn baby, who we'll call Liam, has been diagnosed with sickle cell disease after being screened due to his family's history of the condition. As he grows older, his mother is worried about whether he will be able to engage in regular sports activities. What would be the most suitable advice to give her?

A) Liam can participate, but needs to be careful to avoid dehydration or overly strenuous exercise.

B) Liam should avoid all forms of physical activity to prevent any complications.

C) Liam can participate in sports without any restrictions or precautions.

Question 81: Which illnesses are included in the TORCH syndrome?

A) Tuberculosis, osteoporosis, rubella, cytomegalovirus, herpes simplex

B) Toxoplasmosis, osteoporosis, rubella, cytomegalovirus, herpes simplex

C) Toxoplasmosis, rubella, cytomegalovirus, herpes simplex, other diseases,

Question 82: What should a neonatal intensive care nurse do next after finding that a newborn's blood pressure is 64/40?

A) Record the blood pressure as a normal reading and continue the assessment of the newborn.

B) Immediately start administering blood pressure medication to the newborn.

C) Call for a medical emergency due to the newborn's low blood pressure.

Question 83: In the context of conducting clinical research for evidence-based practice, what factor could potentially undermine its validity?

A) Conducting a double-blind study to avoid bias

B) Including estimated data as well as actual data

C) Using a large sample size for the research

Question 84: What is the maximum percentage of total caloric intake that lipids should represent in a parenteral infusate?

A) 50% of total caloric intake

B) 25% of total caloric intake

C) 75% of total caloric intake

Question 85: In the event of an IV medication extravasation, how many injections of hyaluronidase are typically administered around the edges of the IV insertion site?

A) Seven

B) Three

C) Five

Question 86: What is the mnemonic that can be used as a guide to ensure effective communication during patient handoff?
A) ABCD
B) SBAR
C) EFGH

Question 87: Which electrolyte, when administered, can aid in lowering the risk of neurological impairments in prematurely born infants?
A) Sodium
B) Magnesium
C) Potassium

Question 88: The parents of a newborn, who is currently in the Neonatal Intensive Care Unit, are worried about the placement of an IV in their baby's scalp. How should the nurse alleviate their concerns?
A) The IV is placed in the scalp because it is the most convenient location for the nurse.
B) The IV is positioned in a region with minimal adipose tissue for optimal vein visibility.
C) The IV is placed in the scalp because it causes the least amount of discomfort for the baby.

Question 89: What are the typical symptoms of tracheal stenosis in a newborn baby?
A) Rapid weight gain and excessive sleepiness
B) Biphasic stridor and dyspnea
C) High fever and vomiting

Question 90: In the case of transposition of the great vessels, it can affect the upper and lower vena cavas, the pulmonary artery, and the pulmonary veins. But can you identify which other vessel could be involved in this condition?
A) Aorta
B) Renal Vein
C) Hepatic Artery

Question 91: What is the correct course of action when a newborn, let's call him baby Jack, is delivered from a mother who is currently suffering from varicella at the time of birth?
A) The neonate should be isolated from the mother until her varicella vesicles have crusted over.
B) The neonate should be kept in the same room with the mother to promote bonding.
C) The neonate should be immediately breastfed by the mother to boost his immunity.

Question 92: What is the recommended frequency for changing long-term polyurethane feeding tubes?
A) To the opposite nostril weekly and to a new one monthly
B) To the opposite nostril daily and to a new one weekly
C) To the opposite nostril monthly and to a new one yearly

Question 93: In which category of infants is the occurrence of hypoxic ischemic encephalopathy most frequently observed?
A) Infants with low birth weight
B) Preterm infants
C) Full-term infants

Question 94: What is the term used to describe the least severe type of intraventricular brain hemorrhage in a newborn?
A)A germinal matrix hemorrhage
B) Subdural hemorrhage
C) Subarachnoid hemorrhage

Question 95: Which of the following diseases is a typical example of an autosomal recessive disorder?
A) Huntington's disease
B) Cystic fibrosis
C) Down syndrome

Question 96: What is the primary reason for unclear genitalia in a newborn girl with typical genetics?
A) Turner Syndrome
B) Klinefelter Syndrome
C) Congenital adrenal hyperplasia

Question 97: What guidance should be given to parents to help prevent the occurrence of plagiocephaly, also known as flat head syndrome, in their child?
A) Always keep the infant in a seated position to prevent pressure on the head
B) Always place the infant to sleep on the same side of the head
C) Regularly change the baby's head position and ensure monitored time on their stomach.

Question 98: A newborn baby, who has a central venous line, unexpectedly shows signs of hemodynamic instability, including pulsus paradoxus, slowed heart rate, subdued heart sounds, and a drop in oxygen saturation even with the use of continuous positive airway pressure (CPAP) and heightened oxygen flow. What could these symptoms be indicating?
A) Bronchopulmonary dysplasia
B) Cardiac tamponade
C) Pulmonary embolism

Question 99: What potential conditions could arise from a lack of magnesium in a newborn's diet?

A) Hypocalcemia and hypokalemia

B) Hyperglycemia and hypercalcemia

C) Hypernatremia and hypoglycemia

Question 100: 'What is the signal of an urgent need for intervention due to insufficient uteroplacental function?

A) Early decelerations

B) Accelerations

C) Late decelerations

Question 101: "What is the suggested peak inspiratory pressure (PIP) for a neonate once they have been stabilized on ECMO?"

A) 10 to 14

B) 15 to 22

C) 25 to 30

Question 102: 'Which of the following is NOT considered an early sign of hunger in a newborn?'

A) Persistent crying

B) Rooting reflex

C) Sucking on hands

Question 103: What is the usual impact on the baby when a soon-to-be mother, for instance, Mrs. Michaelson, is given magnesium sulfate as a tocolytic to extend her pregnancy?

A) Increased fetal heart rate and hyperactivity

B) Bradycardia and decreased fetal heart rate variability

C) Increased fetal weight and rapid growth

Question 104: A baby boy, named Jacob, who is 6 days old and was born prematurely at 36 weeks, weighs 6 lbs. He recently had a circumcision procedure. What would be the most suitable dosage of acetaminophen to manage his pain?

A) 1 cc pediatric acetaminophen liquid, orally every 4 hours

B) 2 cc pediatric acetaminophen liquid, orally every 4 hours

C) 1 cc pediatric acetaminophen liquid, orally every 6 hours

Question 105: What does it imply when a newborn is categorized as asymmetrically small for gestational age (SGA)?

A) The neonate is above normal weight for their gestational age.

B) The neonate has both below-normal head circumference and weight.

C) The neonate has normal head circumference but below-normal weight.

Question 106: "What is a condition that may necessitate the use of total parenteral nutrition?"

A) Common Cold

B) Chickenpox

C) Short-gut syndrome

Question 107: At what stage would a child typically begin to exhibit symptoms if they have been diagnosed with late congenital syphilis?

A) Within the first year of life

B) Immediately after birth

C) Post the second year of existence

Question 108: What would be the most suitable course of action if, before administering a tube feeding, the aspirate contains roughly 40% of the previous feeding that hasn't been fully digested?

A) Discard the aspirate and delay the next feeding indefinitely

B) Administer the aspirate back and proceed with the feeding.

C) Immediately administer the next feeding without addressing the undigested aspirate

Question 109: At what stage of gestation does a baby, like little Emma, usually lose her Lanugo?

A) 32 to 36 weeks of gestation

B) 40 to 44 weeks of gestation

C) 20 to 24 weeks of gestation

Question 110: In the Neonatal Intensive Care Unit, a nurse is looking after a newborn baby who hasn't had a bowel movement in the first two days of his life and has been throwing up every time he is fed orally. What could be one of the potential issues with this infant?

A) Hirschsprung's disease

B) Gastroesophageal reflux disease

C) Hypoglycemia

Question 111: "What diagnostic procedure is recommended to steer the therapeutic approach for spontaneous intestinal perforation (FIP)?"

A) Endoscopic biopsy

B) Peritoneal fluid culture

C) Lumbar puncture

Question 112: 'Which nutrients might be excessively lost due to continuous gavage feedings?

A) Vitamins and minerals

B) Fats and calcium

C) Proteins and iron

Question 113: What are the initial steps in the nutritional management of short bowel syndrome following a resection due to necrotizing enterocolitis (NEC)?

A) Immediate introduction of solid foods, hydration, and vitamin supplementation

B) Hydration, electrolyte supplementation, and initiation of parenteral nutrition

C) Fasting, electrolyte supplementation, and initiation of enteral nutrition

Question 114: When a newborn baby is being treated for meningitis with gentamicin, what is the crucial aspect that needs to be closely watched?

A) Skin color

B) Body temperature

C) Renal function

Question 115: "Which baby is at the highest risk of contracting necrotizing enterocolitis?"

A) A premature infant who is formula-fed

B) A full-term infant being breastfed

C) A full-term infant being formula-fed

Question 116: In which scenario does the placenta separate prematurely from the uterine wall, leading to a deprivation of oxygen and nutrients for the fetus?

A) Placenta previa

B) Abruptio placentae

C) Placental insufficiency

Question 117: Where should an intramuscular injection ideally be administered in a preterm or full-term newborn?

A) Deltoid muscle

B) Vastus lateralis/anterolateral thigh

C) Gluteal muscle

Question 118: "What type of gut disorder could potentially develop due to malrotation?"

A) Hemorrhoids

B) Volvulus

C) Appendicitis

Question 119: "When should early oral feedings commence for a newborn who is on tube feedings?"

A) After 1 week

B) Immediately after birth

C) 48 hours

Question 120: In the case of a newborn baby who has been treated with indomethacin due to a patent ductus arteriosus (PDA), which laboratory examinations should be closely observed?

A) Blood glucose level and white blood cell count

B) Liver function and red blood cell count

C) Kidney function and platelet count

Question 121: "In the case of a newborn baby, let's call him Jack, who is suffering from meconium ileus, which condition is he most likely also dealing with?"

A) Down Syndrome

B) Sickle Cell Anemia

C) Cystic fibrosis

Question 122: "What is the condition that impacts nearly 50% of babies born to mothers with diabetes?"

A) Neonatal hypoglycemia

B) Neonatal jaundice

C) Fetal macrosomia

Question 123: In the Neonatal Intensive Care Unit, a premature baby is being nourished through tube feedings until he is ready to try feeding by mouth. What can be done to assist this baby, let's call him Liam, in making the shift from tube feeding to oral feeding?

A) Increase the volume of tube feedings

B) Administer a pacifier for the infant to suck on during tube feedings.

C) Start introducing solid foods immediately

Question 124: "At what age is a newborn baby typically able to raise their head while lying on their stomach?"

A) At birth

B) 3 months

C) 6 weeks

Question 125: At what stage of hypoxic-ischemic encephalopathy (HIE) might a patient, let's say Thomas, potentially experience seizures?

A) Stage 1

B) Stage 2

C) Stage 3

Question 126: "What could be a severe consequence related to meconium aspiration in a newborn baby?"

A) Gastroesophageal reflux disease (GERD)

B) PPHN (persistent pulmonary hypertension of the newborn)

C) Congenital hypothyroidism

Question 127: What is the primary cause of nosocomial (hospital-acquired) infections in full-term newborns?

A) Staphylococcus aureus

B) Streptococcus pneumoniae

C) Escherichia coli

Question 128: What classification grade would be assigned to an intraventricular hemorrhage that has extended into 10% to 40% of the lateral ventricles, but has not caused any significant dilation?

A) II

B) I

C) III

Question 129: What is the typical treatment approach for a newborn, suffering from mixed type Apnea of Prematurity (AOP)?

A) Administration of Caffeine and usage of CPAP

B) Use of anticonvulsants and ventilator support

C) Administration of antibiotics only

Question 130: What is the comparison between the protein content in colostrum and that in mature human milk?

A) The protein content is lower in colostrum than in mature milk.

B) The protein content in colostrum and mature human milk is the same.

C) The protein content is higher in colostrum than in mature milk.

Question 131: "What could be a potential reason for a newborn baby to experience direct hyperbilirubinemia?"

A) Normal newborn jaundice

B) Extrahepatic biliary atresia

C) Excessive milk intake

Question 132: "What is typically the primary reason for direct hyperbilirubinemia in a newborn baby?"

A) Inadequate breast milk intake

B) Liver immaturity

C) Overexposure to sunlight

Question 133: "In which gestational age group are neonates primarily affected by Intraventricular hemorrhage (IVH)?"

A) <<32 weeks

B) 35-37 weeks

C) 40-42 weeks

Question 134: "What is the body's automatic reaction to stress?"

A) Sweating profusely

B) Flushing

C) Fainting

Question 135 : "In a newborn baby, what is typically the primary reason for the occurrence of pneumothorax?"

A) Congenital heart disease

B) Hypoglycemia

C) Respiratory distress syndrome

Question 136: "What is the recommended vitamin to administer to newborns who are susceptible to developing bronchopulmonary dysplasia?"

A) Vitamin D

B) Vitamin C

C) Vitamin A

Question 137: What is the most effective method to communicate with a patient, let's call her Maria, and her family who do not speak English?

A) Ensure the presence of an interpreter proficient in medical terminology.

B) Speak slowly and loudly in English

C) Use hand gestures and body language to communicate

Question 138: A baby boy, newly born, has been found to have neonatal testicular torsion, resulting in one testicle being beyond repair, while the other remains unaffected. His parents are concerned about whether this condition will impact his ability to have children in the future. What would be the most suitable reply to their query?

A) The unaffected testicle will also eventually become damaged due to this condition.

B) This condition will definitely lead to infertility in the future.

C)The likelihood of enduring fertility complications due to this condition is extremely minimal.

Question 139: "Which method is not advised for giving naloxone (Narcan) to babies?"

A) Intramuscular

B) Intravenous

C) Endotracheal

Question 140: "What is the most frequent heart irregularity associated with Trisomy 18?"

A) Ventricular fibrillation

B) Atrial-septal defect

C) Sinus bradycardia

Question 141: 'What is typically linked with the occurrence of neonatal abstinence syndrome (NAS)?'

A) NAS is generally linked to the neonate's exposure to loud noises and bright lights.

B) NAS may result from the neonate's iatrogenic exposure to opiates intended for sedation or analgesia.

C) NAS is typically caused by the mother's consumption of spicy foods during pregnancy.

Question 142: For which condition would it be advised to either provide a private room or group together patients suffering from the same infection, in a medical setting?

A) Asthma

B) Common Cold

C) Gastroenteritis

Question 143: "What approach should be employed to nourish a prematurely born baby, like little Emma, who has a feeble sucking reflex?"

A) Oral feeding using a bottle

B) Gavage feeding

C) Intravenous feeding

Question 144: "Which medical condition might necessitate the continuous use of total parenteral nutrition?"
A) Common cold
B) Short bowel syndrome
C) Chickenpox

Question 145: What is the term for the model of care in the Neonatal Intensive Care Unit (NICU) where neonates are looked after by a collaborative team comprising of nurses, doctors, respiratory therapists, and occupational therapists?
A) Interprofessional Practice
B) Single Professional Practice
C) Independent Practice

Question 146: What is typically the primary reason for experiencing discomfort in the nipples for a mother who is breastfeeding?
A) Mother's stress levels
B) Consumption of spicy foods
C) Inappropriate positioning and latching on

Question 147: Can you explain what is meant by the term "patent ductus arteriosus"?
A) A blockage in the superior vena cava
B) An opening between the pulmonary and aortic arteries
C) A closure of the ventricular septum

Question 148: What would be the most accurate description of a situation where the parents of a newborn baby in the Neonatal Intensive Care Unit are present at every infant care meeting and contribute to all care-related decisions?
A) Shared decision making
B) Medical team dominance in decision making
C) Parental dominance in decision making

Question 149: What is the maximum speed at which fat emulsions for parenteral nutrition should be given?
A) 0.5 g/kg/hr
B) 0.2 g/kg/hr
C) 1.0 g/kg/hr

Question 150: "What additional evaluations should be conducted for a newborn, like baby Mia, who has been diagnosed with an omphalocele?"
A) Immediate surgery
B) No further evaluations needed
C) Associated anomalies

Question 151: What could be the possible outcome if the glucose intake of a newborn, who is on parenteral nutrition, is decreased too rapidly?
A) Reactive hypoglycemia
B) Hypernatremia
C) Increased metabolic rate

Question 152: What is the procedure in neonatal care where the use of an opioid is deemed suitable to alleviate pain?
A) Performing a routine physical examination on the neonate
B) Administration or extraction of a peripherally inserted central catheter (PICC line).
C) Administering a standard immunization shot

Question 153: Which of the following conditions is a type of congenital heart disease that results in cyanosis?
A) Acute bronchitis
B) Asthma
C) Hypoplastic left heart syndrome

Question 154: A neonatal intensive care nurse is assessing a newborn baby. The baby is exhibiting signs of respiratory distress, such as retractions during breathing and a low grunting noise accompanying his fast breaths. What could be the most probable diagnosis for these symptoms?
A) Meconium aspiration syndrome
B) Hypoglycemia
C) Neonatal jaundice

Question 155: Can you explain the distinction between an omphalocele and a gastroschisis?
A) An omphalocele is a condition where the abdominal contents protrude through the umbilicus, and a gastroschisis is a condition where the abdominal contents protrude through a defect in the abdominal wall.
B) An omphalocele is characterized by the protrusion of abdominal contents through the umbilicus, whereas in gastroschisis, the abdominal organs lack a protective membrane cover.
C) An omphalocele and a gastroschisis are both conditions where the abdominal contents protrude through the umbilicus, but in a gastroschisis, the abdominal contents are covered by a membrane.

Question 156: When a nurse observes a subtle bluish discoloration around the mouth of a newborn baby, what should be the initial course of action?
A) Immediately administer oxygen without further assessment.
B)Examine the infant's entire body for signs of cyanosis in the extremities and check for retractions or other indications of respiratory distress.

C) Ignore the discoloration as it is a common occurrence in newborns.

Question 157: 'If a quad screen test reveals decreased levels of AFP, elevated hCG, reduced uE^3, and increased INH-A, what condition does this typically indicate?**
A) Neural Tube Defects
B) Trisomy 18
C) Trisomy 21

Question 158: "What should be the proportion of cerebrospinal glucose level in comparison to the plasma glucose level?"
A) 60% to 70%
B) 80% to 90%
C) 30% to 40%

Question 159: What condition is a newborn with periventricular leukomalacia more likely to develop?**
A) Diabetes
B) Asthma
C) Cerebral palsy

Question 160: A newborn baby, who arrived prematurely at 31 weeks and showed signs of respiratory distress syndrome, was immediately put on CPAP post-birth. However, within a few hours, the baby required a FiO2 of 0.40. What does this suggest?**
A) The baby is experiencing normal oxygen levels
B) The baby is experiencing CPAP failure
C) The baby is showing signs of improvement

Question 161: "Which baby is at the highest risk of contracting necrotizing enterocolitis?"
A) A full-term infant being breastfed
B) A premature infant being breastfed
C) A premature infant being formula fed

Question 162: During which trimester is the unborn baby most susceptible to developing birth defects if the mother contracts toxoplasmosis?**
A) Second
B) First
C) Third

Question 163: After the delivery, it is recommended that neonates with a very low birth weight (VLBW) should initiate skin-to-skin contact, also known as kangaroo care, with their mother within what timeframe?**
A) 60 minutes
B) Immediately after birth
C) Within 24 hours

Question 164: What should be the subsequent course of action if a new tracheostomy tube cannot be inserted into a newborn after two attempts?**
A) Try a tube that is a half size smaller
B) Continue to attempt insertion with the same size tube
C) Use a tube that is a half size larger

Question 165: "What type of parasitic infection can potentially be caused by the excrement of domestic felines?"
A) Malaria
B) Leishmaniasis
C) Toxoplasmosis

Question 166: Considering that only a tenth of the iron from formula is absorbed, what proportion of iron from breast milk would be absorbed?**
A) 60%
B) 50%
C) 80%

Question 167: In a scenario where a newborn baby, weighing 3 kg, is diagnosed with isoimmune hemolytic anemia and requires an exchange transfusion, what would be the volume of each aliquot that needs to be taken out and then replaced?**
A) 30 mL per aliquot
B) 20 mL per aliquot
C) 10 mL per aliquot

Question 168: "What could be the main reason behind the occurrence of central cyanosis?"
A) Minor skin infection
B) Heart failure
C) Dehydration

Question 169: "Which of the following options best describes a method of providing care that incorporates socioemotional aspects?"
A) Ignoring the infant's crying
B) Leaving the infant alone for long periods of time
C) Engaging in play activities with the baby

Question 170: "In the case of an infant being breastfed, which vitamin is typically required as a supplement?"
A) Vitamin C
B) Vitamin D
C) Vitamin A

Question 171: What is the recommended preventive measure for newborns, like baby Michael, who are susceptible to low blood sugar levels?**
A) Limiting fluid intake

B) Delayed feedings

C) Early feedings

Question 172: In the Neonatal Intensive Care Unit, a nurse is looking after a newborn baby. The baby hasn't had any bowel movement in the initial 48 hours after birth and shows signs of vomiting each time oral feeding is tried. What could be one of the potential health issues the baby is facing?

A) Gastroesophageal reflux disease

B) Neonatal jaundice

C) Hirschsprung's disease

Question 173: What condition is a hypothermic newborn more likely to develop?

A) Hyperthermia

B) Hypoglycemia

C) Hyperglycemia

Question 174: "What is the main reason for skin deterioration in newborn babies?"

A) Adhesive

B) Excessive bathing

C) Exposure to sunlight

Question 175: A newborn baby, born prematurely at 29 weeks, has been tested and the following arterial blood gas values have been recorded: pH - 7.36, pCO2 - 52, HCO3 - 30. What do these values suggest?

A) Compensated respiratory acidosis

B) Uncompensated respiratory alkalosis

C) Metabolic alkalosis

Question 176: What is the likelihood of a newborn, whose parents are both carriers of the sickle cell trait, developing sickle cell disease, considering it's an autosomal recessive condition?

A) 75%

B) 50%

C) 25%

Question 177: What genetic disorder is commonly associated with an atrioventricular septal defect, or in milder cases, a ventricular septal defect, that a neonatal intensive care nurse might encounter?

A) Marfan syndrome

B) Turner syndrome

C) Down syndrome

Question 178: A phone call is received by the nurse from the grandmother of a patient, let's name him Timmy. She has been unsuccessful in contacting Timmy's parents as they have been constantly by his side. She is seeking an update on Timmy's health status. What would be the most appropriate response from the nurse?

A) Ignore the call and continue with your duties without informing Timmy's parents about the call.

B) Provide the grandmother with a detailed update on Timmy's health status, including his current condition and treatment plan.

C) Inform her that it's not permissible to divulge any information, however, you will notify the parents about her call and request them to get in touch with her.

Question 179: How would you compare the PaCO2 level in the venous umbilical cord blood to the PaCO2 level in the arterial umbilical cord blood?

A) Higher

B) Lower

C) Equal

Question 180: In the Neonatal Intensive Care Unit, for how long should a newborn be exclusively fed with colostrum?

A) 3 to 4 days

B) 1 to 2 days

C) 5 to 6 days

Question 181: What is the best approach to mitigate discomfort when collecting a capillary blood sample by piercing a newborn's heel?

A) Administer a mild sedative to the newborn before the heel lance

B) Apply a cold pack to the heel prior to the heel lance

C) Provide a pacifier dipped in sucrose for 2 minutes before the heel lance

Question 182: A newborn baby, diagnosed with a neural tube defect, presents a significant myelomeningocele at the lower part of their spine. What should be the first course of action in this scenario?

A) Apply warm saline-soaked gauze and plastic wrap over the exposed tissue

B) Administer high doses of antibiotics immediately

C) Perform immediate surgery to close the defect

Question 183: "In the event of pulmonary stenosis not receiving treatment, which part of the heart would be most impacted?"

A) Right ventricle

B) Left ventricle

C) Left atrium

Question 184: A premature baby girl, born at 30 weeks, is ready to be discharged from the NICU. She's been doing well with bottle feedings and has managed to nurse successfully twice. Her mother is keen on continuing to breastfeed her at home. What would be a crucial topic to incorporate into the discharge planning and education at this point?

A) Switching to formula feeding

B) The importance of using pacifiers

C) Lactation consult

Question 185: "Does Turner's syndrome predominantly occur in newborn boys or girls?"

A) It affects both males and females equally.

B) It affects males only.

C) Only female newborns are affected

Question 186: What is the main reason for adding breast milk fortifiers to the human breast milk given to premature newborns?

A) To enhance the taste of the breast milk for the newborn

B) To change the color of the breast milk for aesthetic purposes

C) Human breast milk is deficient in protein content.

Question 187: In the case of a newborn, let's say baby James, who is suspected of having a right-to-left shunt due to an open ductus arteriosus, where should the electrodes be placed for monitoring the transcutaneous carbon dioxide levels?

A) The right shoulder and lower abdomen

B) The left shoulder and upper abdomen

C) The left leg and right arm

Question 188: What is the purpose of replacing lactose with glucose polymers in infant feedings?

A) It increases the caloric content of formulas.

B) It reduces the osmotic concentration of formulas.

C) It improves the taste of the formula.

Question 189: 'If the parents of a newborn baby boy, let's call him Ethan, have decided against circumcision, what should be part of the care guidelines provided to them?'

A) The foreskin should be left as it is, without any cleaning or drying.

B) The foreskin has to be completely retracted for cleaning. Dry the area well.

C) The foreskin should be partially retracted for cleaning and the area should be left moist.

Question 190: "In the context of significant drug-to-drug interactions (DDIs) in newborns, which medication is most likely to be involved?"

A) Fentanyl

B) Ibuprofen

C) Paracetamol

Question 191: For neonates who are 34 weeks or older and require nasal continuous positive airway pressure (CPAP), what should the initial attempt include when transitioning to breastfeeding?

A) 10 minutes attempt at sucking a partially pumped breast

B) Immediate transition to bottle feeding

C) 5 minutes attempt at sucking a fully pumped breast

Question 192: "Which condition is associated with a chromosomal abnormality in chromosome 22?"

A) DiGeorge Syndrome

B) Down Syndrome

C) Turner Syndrome

Question 193: "What condition could be suggested by the pattern observed in a newborn's ECG tracing?"

A) Hypoglycemia

B) Neonatal jaundice

C) Supraventricular tachycardia

Question 194: What is typically necessary for a newborn baby to quickly achieve a steady state of a medication's plasma concentration?

A) An initial high dose

B) A reduced dose

C) No medication at all

Question 195: At what point does the breast milk of a preterm baby start to have similar characteristics as that of a full-term baby?

A) 10 to 12 weeks

B) 5 to 7 weeks

C) 1 to 2 weeks

Question 196: What is the implication if the discharge from a newly formed colostomy is measured at 4 mL/kg/hour?

A) The colostomy is functioning normally

B) The patient needs immediate surgery

C) Initiation of fluid replenishment is necessary.

Question 197: In the context of neonatal resuscitation, at what heart rate threshold should a neonate, who is receiving sufficient and effective ventilation, begin to receive chest compressions (cardiac massage)?

A) 60 bpm

B) 80 bpm

C) 100 bpm

Question 198: What are the clinical signs associated with renal vein thrombosis in newborns?

A) Hypertension

B) Thrombocytopenia

C) Hyperglycemia

Question 199: What is the preferred method of treatment for a pregnant woman, let's call her Mary, who has been diagnosed with primary syphilis?

A) Doxycycline, 100 mg orally twice a day for 14 days

B) Azithromycin, single dose of 1 g orally

C) Benzathine penicillin, one 2.4-million-unit injection

Question 200: 'What is a significant risk factor that can lead to the development of severe hyperbilirubinemia?'

A) Prolonged gestation period

B) Cephalohematoma

C) High birth weight

Question 201: What is the primary purpose of administering oral sucrose to newborns?

A) To increase body weight

B) Pain relief

C) To stimulate appetite

Question 202: In which category of infants is the occurrence of hypoxic ischemic encephalopathy more frequently observed?

A) Full-term infants

B) Infants with high birth weight

C) Premature infants

Question 203: In the context of nursing, can you identify an instance of nonmaleficence from the options given?

A) Ignoring a patient's request for assistance with personal hygiene.

B) Administering pain medication to a patient prior to conducting wound care.

C) Administering a medication without checking the patient's allergies first.

Question 204: What is the preferred initial diagnostic procedure when a newborn, let's say baby Charles, is suspected to have a lower bowel obstruction?

A) An echocardiogram

B) A contrast enema

C) A cranial ultrasound

Question 205: What medical condition might a newborn baby develop due to Rh factor incompatibility?

A) Down Syndrome

B) Cystic Fibrosis

C) Hydrops fetalis

Question 206: What is a significant benefit of employing the Teach-Back method when providing education to patients and their families?

A) To reduce the time spent on patient education

B) To confirm the comprehensive understanding of imparted information.

C) To avoid the necessity for follow-up appointments

Question 207: In what situation would the KleihauerBetke test be beneficial?

A) A 32-year-old non-pregnant female experiencing severe headaches and blurred vision.

B) A pregnant woman of 29 years, at her 26th week of gestation, experiencing abdominal discomfort after tumbling down a long staircase.

C) A 45-year-old male patient experiencing chest pain after a strenuous workout.

Question 208: In the context of the ABCs of neonatal resuscitation, which includes airway, breathing, and circulation, what action should the nurse take to stimulate breathing in the newborn?

A) Administer high-dose epinephrine

B) Stimulate the neonate's back and limbs.

C) Immediately perform chest compressions

Question 209: In emergency scenarios, which neonatal intervention necessitates the informed consent of a parent or legal guardian?

A) Administration of routine vaccinations

B) Routine physical examination

C) Blood transfusion

Question 210: 'How does the insensible water loss (IWL) in newborns placed under radiant warmers in incubators compare to the standard IWL in neonates?

A) No change in IWL

B) Increased IWL by 40% to 50%

C) Decreased IWL by 20% to 30%

Question 211: "What is the primary reason for respiratory distress syndrome in a newborn?"

A) Congenital heart disease

B) Neonatal sepsis

C)Newborn Transient Tachypnea

Question 212: "What is the approximate capacity of a newborn's stomach on their very first day of life?"

A) 15 to 20 mL

B) 30 to 35 mL

C) 5 to 7 mL

Question 213: In the Neonatal Intensive Care Unit, a preterm baby, let's call him Sam, has a G-tube in place. The nurse is beginning his routine feeding, but encounters a problem - the formula isn't flowing properly and is accumulating in the tube. What should the nurse's subsequent course of action be?

A) Proceed with a 5-10 cc warm water flush in the G-tube, and if resistance is encountered, perform aspiration and additional flushing

B) Remove the G-tube and insert a new one

C) Increase the speed of the formula flow to force it through the tube

Question 214: What is the medical term for the swelling of the head that extends beyond the suture lines in a newborn?

A) Caput succedaneum

B) Cephalohematoma

C) Hydrocephalus

Question 215: What is the standard temperature setting for both electric and disposable warming mattresses in neonatal care?

A) 120 °F

B) 85 °F

C) 100 °F

Question 216: In the case of a premature infant, what condition would necessitate the use of parenteral nutrition?

A) Infants with a birth weight of more than 2500 g

B) Infants with a birth weight of 2000 to 2500 g

C) Infants with extremely low birth weight (below 1500 g)

Question 217: "What health complication might arise in a newborn baby, such as baby Mia, due to Rh factor discrepancy?"

A) Hydrops fetalis

B) Congenital heart disease

C) Cystic fibrosis

Question 218: "Which among the following options is typically NOT a hurdle to the interaction between a parent and their newborn?"

A) The newborn's critical health condition

B) Well-educated parents

C) Limited visitation hours in the NICU

Question 219: For a newborn baby experiencing respiratory distress, what is the optimal time period for administering surfactant?

A) Within 1 hour of birth

B) After 48 hours of birth

C) Within 24 hours of birth

Question 220: "What is the most common timeframe for the onset of postpartum depression to occur?"

A) Six months postpartum

B) Immediately after delivery

C) Four weeks postpartum

Question 221: Which of the following scenarios best illustrates the concept of beneficence in nursing practice?

A) Ignoring a patient's request for pain medication because they have a history of drug abuse

B) Assisting patients in performing their ADLs when self-execution is not possible.

C) Refusing to provide care to a patient because of their infectious disease status

Question 222: In the Neonatal Intensive Care Unit, a newborn baby named Ethan consistently turns his head in response to the sound of a monitor alarm. However, after hearing this sound repeatedly throughout the day, he eventually stops reacting to it. What is the medical term for this absence of response?

A) Habituation

B) Sensory deprivation

C) Sensory overload

Question 223: What are the typical signs that a patient might exhibit if they abruptly stop taking their beta-blocker medication?

A) Normal blood pressure, normal heart rate, cardiac dysrhythmias, no tremors, and sweating

B) Hypotension, decreased heart rate, normal cardiac rhythm, no tremors, and no sweating

C)Elevated blood pressure, accelerated heart rhythm, heart rhythm disorders, shivering, and perspiration.

Question 224: "In the case of Hirschsprung disease, which part of the body is primarily impacted?"

A) The heart

B) The lungs

C) The colon

Question 225: What is the recommendation of the American Academy of Pediatrics (AAP) for managing gastroesophageal reflux in preterm newborns?

A) No specific treatment

B) Surgical intervention

C) Administration of antacids

Question 226: What is the primary reason for respiratory acidosis to occur?

A) Hypoventilation

B) Hypertension

C) Overhydration

Question 227: A newborn baby has been diagnosed with galactosemia. His mother, let's call her Mrs. Smith, is curious to know if breastfeeding is still an option for her. What would be the most appropriate response to her query?

A) Mrs. Smith can breastfeed her baby without any issues as galactosemia does not affect breastfeeding.
B) Mrs. Smith can breastfeed her baby, but she needs to limit the frequency to avoid overconsumption of galactose.
C) Mrs. Smith will not be able to breastfeed because of the risk of ingesting galactose in the milk.

Question 228: "What type of skin condition could potentially indicate the presence of neurofibromatosis?"
A) Psoriasis
B) Café au lait spots
C) Vitiligo

Question 229: In a scenario where a newborn baby, let's call him Baby Charles, is diagnosed with hydrops fetalis and is experiencing respiratory distress along with uneven breathing sounds, what medical condition is most likely indicated?
A) Bronchopulmonary dysplasia
B) Congenital heart disease
C) Pneumothorax

Question 230: In a situation where a teenage mother of a newborn baby is constantly accompanied by her own mother - the baby's grandmother, who seems to be in control. To whom should the nurse direct her updates about the baby's health status and inquiries about care decisions?
A) The mother of the newborn
B) The baby's grandmother
C) The hospital's pediatrician

Question 231: "Which medication from the list below is not recommended for treating a baby experiencing breathing difficulties?"
A) Formoterol (Perforomist)
B) Budesonide (Pulmicort)
C) Albuterol (Proventil)

Question 232: What could be a potential ultrasound discovery during pregnancy that might suggest the presence of esophageal atresia?
A) Polyhydramnios
B) Decreased amniotic fluid levels
C) Normal placental position

Question 233: 'What is a typical symptom of hydrocephalus in a newborn baby?'
A) Sunsetting sign
B) Rapid weight gain
C) Dry skin

Question 234: "What indicates a bond or connection being formed? "
A) The parent ignores the crying infant.
B) The parent immediately picks up and comforts the crying infant.
C) The parent leaves the room when the infant starts crying.

Question 235: What potential risk could an intubated newborn baby, who is experiencing hyperventilation, face?
A) Metabolic acidosis
B) Respiratory acidosis
C) Respiratory alkalosis

Question 236: "What is the primary function of stay sutures after a tracheostomy procedure has been performed?"
A) To close the wound immediately after surgery
B) Maintain an open stoma
C) To stop bleeding from the surgical site

Question 237: "What role does the pulmonary surfactant play in a newborn's body?"
A) Enhances the production of red blood cells
B) Inhibits the collapse of alveoli in the neonate.
C) Stimulates the production of breast milk

Question 238: In the Neonatal Intensive Care Unit, a preterm baby, who we'll call Baby Jake, has been fitted with a G-tube. The nurse is about to begin his regular feeding, but notices that the formula isn't flowing properly and is instead accumulating in the tube. What should the nurse do next?
A) Continue with the feeding, the formula will eventually flow through the tube.
B)Administer a 5-10 cc warm water flush through the G-tube, and if resistance is encountered, attempt aspiration and further flushing.
C) Remove the G-tube and replace it with a new one.

Question 239: What is the best course of action for a newborn named Lily, who has a feeding tube and is undergoing CPAP treatment, if she starts to show signs of abdominal bloating?
A) Insert an orogastric tube of 8-French size or larger.
B) Increase the feeding tube flow rate
C) Remove the CPAP treatment immediately

Question 240: In the case where a patient, let's call her Jane, is believed to have placenta previa, which procedure is strictly not recommended?
A) Ultrasound scan
B) Digital vaginal exam
C) Blood tests

Question 241: In the case of chronic lung disease or bronchopulmonary dysplasia leading to bronchospasm, which medication would be the preferred treatment option?
A) Amoxicillin
B) Albuterol
C) Ibuprofen

Question 242: What is the most suitable course of action for a neonate, who has been exposed to drugs and often brings up his feedings?
A) Feed the neonate lying flat on his back immediately after feeding.
B) Feed the neonate less frequently, but with larger amounts.
C) Hold the neonate upright for 15 to 20 minutes after feeding.

Question 243: Which condition is known to elevate the chances of developing pulmonary hypoplasia?
A) Hyperglycemia
B) Oligohydramnios
C) Hypocalcemia

Question 244: "Which statement about anticipatory grieving is not true?"
A) It is a normal part of the grieving process to anticipate the loss of a loved one, even if that loss is not imminent.
B) It is typical for parents to maintain continuous emotional disconnection from their infant well beyond the point where the infant demonstrates signs of recovery or survival.
C) Anticipatory grieving can help parents prepare emotionally for the potential loss of their infant.

Question 245: What is the probable diagnosis for a mother, say Mrs. Danielson, who experiences episodes of emotional instability, frequent crying, and feelings of worry a few days after giving birth?
A) Postpartum psychosis
B) Postpartum depression
C) Postpartum blues

Question 246: A nurse is attending to a newborn diagnosed with spina bifida. The baby's mother, whom we'll call Mrs. Smith, is worried that a tumble she took two weeks prior to giving birth might be the reason for her baby's condition. What would be the most appropriate response to her concern?

A) "Spina bifida is usually caused by a combination of genetic and environmental factors, but it is not related to any physical trauma during pregnancy."
B) "The fall could have triggered the development of spina bifida in the baby."
C) Spina bifida's formation occurs within the initial month of gestation, so the fall she experienced weeks before delivery is unrelated.

Question 247: In the Neonatal Intensive Care Unit, a prematurely born baby girl, who has a nasogastric drain, presents the following arterial blood gas results: pH 7.5, HCO329, pCO237. What type of acid-base imbalance can be inferred from these values?
A) Metabolic alkalosis
B) Metabolic acidosis
C) Respiratory alkalosis

Question 248: "Which heart disorder is typically associated with symptoms such as feeble peripheral pulses and cold limbs?"
A) Ventricular Septal Defect
B) Atrial Septal Defect
C) Hypoplastic left heart syndrome

Question 249: "On what factors does the progression of proprioception rely?"
A) Visual and auditory senses
B) Movement and touch
C) Taste and smell

Question 250: What does it signify if a newborn's umbilical cord shows signs of green or yellow tinge?
A) Meconium staining
B) Indication of a bacterial infection
C) Sign of jaundice

Question 251: "What type of parasitic infection can be caused by the excrement of domestic felines?"
A) Malaria
B) Toxoplasmosis
C) Leishmaniasis

Question 252: If the parents of a newborn, who is showing signs of improvement, appear to be growing more anxious and repeatedly inquire if their baby is on the verge of death, what would be the most suitable response?
A) "You need to stop worrying so much, your baby is getting better."
B) "Can you tell me what you understand about your baby's condition?"
C) "I think you are overreacting; your baby is not on the verge of death."

Question 253: In the case of a newborn baby with malrotation, what type of acid-base imbalance would suggest the presence of volvulus?

A) Metabolic alkalosis

B) Respiratory alkalosis

C) Metabolic acidosis

Question 254: What should be the maintained FiO2 level with noninvasive or mechanical ventilation for a preterm newborn in order to avoid oxygen toxicity?

A) 0.70

B) <<0.50

C) 0.80

Question 255: When it comes to the positioning of an infant in a car seat, where should the uppermost part of the chest clips ideally be situated, as per the advice given to parents?

A) At armpit level

B) At the level of the belly button

C) At the level of the neck

Question 256: The arterial blood gas (ABG) results of a newborn baby, whom we'll call Baby Jane, are as follows: pH is 7.24, PaCO2 is 56 mmHg, HCO3- is 25 mEq/L, PaO2 is 57 mmHg, and the base excess is -4. What do these readings suggest about Baby Jane's condition?

A) Metabolic alkalosis

B) Respiratory acidosis

C) Respiratory alkalosis

Question 257: What is the best course of action to manage hyperbilirubinemia related to breastfeeding?

A) Increase the frequency of breastfeedings

B) Give the infant sugar water instead of breastfeeding

C) Decrease the frequency of breastfeedings

Question 258: "Which factor would contribute the most to the increased loss of insensible water?"

A) Infants of smaller size and premature gestational age

B) Increased fluid intake

C) Increased ambient temperature

Question 259: A newborn baby, displaying features such as extra fingers or toes (polydactyly), closely spaced eyes, a small jaw (micrognathia), a smaller than normal head size (microcephaly), a cleft lip, and a single crease across the palm. Which type of trisomy do these symptoms suggest?

A) Trisomy 18

B) Trisomy 13

C) Trisomy 21

Question 260: 'Which test is most effective in distinguishing between cardiac and respiratory origins of central cyanosis?

A) Echocardiogram

B) Spirometry test

C) Hyperoxia test

Question 261: "Which electrolyte has been found to decrease the risk of neurological issues in prematurely born babies?"

A) Calcium

B) Magnesium

C) Potassium

Question 262: What is the daily rate at which feeding volumes should be increased for most preterm newborns, after starting with minimal enteral feedings?

A) 10 to 20 mL/kg/day

B) 50 to 60 mL/kg/day

C) 30 to 40 mL/kg/day

Question 263: "What could be the potential impact on the heart when muscle relaxants like pancuronium bromide, vecuronium, or rocuronium are administered to newborns on mechanical ventilation?"

A) Bradycardia

B) No change in heart rate

C) Tachycardia

Question 264: A pregnant woman, let's call her Jane, is experiencing symptoms such as a high temperature, an elevated white blood cell count (more than 15,000 per mm3), rapid heart rate in both her and her unborn child, and a discharge from her vagina that appears to be filled with pus. Can you identify the medical condition that these symptoms typically indicate?

A) Pre-eclampsia

B) Gestational Diabetes

C) Chorioamnionitis

Question 265: What does a score of 3 signify on the Infant-Driven Feeding Scales (IDFS) - Readiness Score Description?

A) The neonate is ready for oral feedings

B) The neonate requires tube feeding.

C) The neonate can be breastfed directly

Question 266: In the context of kangaroo care, what is the appropriate positioning for a newborn baby?

A) Unclothed (diaper is acceptable), placed horizontally on caregiver's bare chest

B) The neonate is positioned vertically, bare except for a diaper, on the caregiver's exposed chest.'

C) Fully clothed, placed horizontally on the caregiver's lap

Question 267: A nurse receives instructions to administer dobutamine via an intravenous route. What should she be aware of regarding this procedure?

A) This should be given through an oral route.

B) This should be given through a nasal route.

C) This must be administered through a central line.

Question 268: "Which mineral level frequently drops following the intravenous administration of Lasix?"

A) Iron

B) Calcium

C) Zinc

Question 269: What should a neonatal intensive care nurse do next after finding out that the blood pressure of a newborn baby, let's call him baby Jack, is 64/40?

A) Call for a medical emergency as the blood pressure is too low.

B) Immediately administer medication to increase the baby's blood pressure.

C)Log the blood pressure as a standard measurement and proceed with the newborn's evaluation.

Question 270: What is a characteristic symptom of tracheomalacia in a newborn baby?

A) Excessive sleepiness and lethargy

B) Increased heart rate and high blood pressure

C) Noisy breathing and dyspnea when crying or feeding

Question 271: "What is the most frequent negative impact on a newborn due to a Cesarean section?"

A) Delayed lactation

B) Respiratory distress

C) Increased immunity

Question 272: In the case of transposition of the great vessels, it can affect the superior and inferior vena cavas, the pulmonary artery, and the pulmonary veins. Can you identify the other potential vessel that could be involved in this condition?

A) Aorta

B) Carotid Artery

C) Coronary Artery

Question 273: "What is the most frequently observed blood-related symptom in cases of preeclampsia?"

A) Polycythemia

B) Hyperglycemia

C) Thrombocytopenia

Question 274: "What is the primary objective of quality improvement in a medical setting?"

A) To reduce the workload of the medical staff

B) To enact precise modifications that yield quantifiable enhancements for a patient cohort.

C) To increase the revenue of the medical facility

Question 275: What could be a potential outcome if coarctation of the aorta is not addressed in a timely manner?

A) Development of superior vena cava syndrome

B) Spontaneous resolution of the condition

C) Congestive heart failure

Question 276: What is the rate at which High-frequency ventilation (HFV) administers small tidal volumes?

A) 150/min

B) 200/min

C) 75/min

Question 277: In a scenario where the parents of a newborn, who reside in a different location, are maintaining contact with the medical team through video calls to foster bonding, what should be the primary concern of the nurse?

A) The infant's reactions and progress

B) The convenience of the parents' schedule

C) The quality of the video call

Question 278: What is the typical duration of a sleep cycle for a newborn baby?

A) 30 to 40 minutes

B) 50 to 60 minutes

C) 90 to 120 minutes

Question 279: What would be the likely diagnosis for a newborn baby girl, who presents with a webbed neck (cystic hygromata), low-set ears, and nipples that are spaced widely apart?

A) Down syndrome

B) Turner syndrome

C) Klinefelter syndrome

Question 280: A woman named Linda had to go through an unplanned Cesarean section at 32 weeks of pregnancy. Now, she is constantly experiencing nightmares and showing signs of hypervigilance while her newborn is in the Neonatal Intensive Care Unit (NICU). What could these symptoms suggest?

A) Adjustment disorder

B) Posttraumatic stress disorder

C) Postpartum depression

Question 281: "Among the listed congenital heart abnormalities, which one is recognized as a condition causing cyanosis?"

A) Atrial Septal Defect

B) Tetralogy of Fallot

C) Ventricular Septal Defect

Question 282: What is the threshold temperature for defining hyperthermia in terms of core body temperature?

A) 36.5 °C

B) 37.5 °C

C) 38.5 °C

Question 283: During the initial 72 hours of a newborn being treated with extracorporeal membrane oxygenation (ECMO), what should be the maintained level of platelet count in the blood?

A) >100,000 per mm3

B) <50,000 per mm3

C) 70,000-80,000 per mm3

Question 284: What is the third factor, alongside dryness and erythema, that the Neonatal Skin Condition Score takes into consideration?

A) Breakdown

B) Heart rate

C) Temperature

Question 285: What should be the expected decrease in bilirubin levels in a newborn, named Lucy, after she has undergone 24 hours of phototherapy for hyperbilirubinemia treatment?

A) 50% to 60%

B) 30% to 40%

C) 10% to 20%

Question 286: An infant boy, who we'll call Noah, was delivered prematurely at 35 weeks. His birth came after his mother endured 26 hours of labor, during which she had a fever of 38.5 °C. An intrauterine fetal monitoring device was used during her labor. Now, an hour after his birth, Noah is showing signs of respiratory distress and cyanosis, his body temperature is a mere 36 °C, and he appears extremely lethargic. What could be the most probable reason for Noah's current state?

A) Neonatal hypoglycemia

B) Neonatal jaundice

C) Streptococcus Group B infection

Question 287: "Which method is not advised for giving naloxone (Narcan) to newborns?"

A) Intramuscular

B) Intravenous

C) Endotracheal

Question 288: While providing a blood transfusion to a premature baby named Lily who is suffering from anemia, what symptom might indicate that she is having a possible transfusion reaction?

A) Increased appetite

B) Rapid hair growth

C) Tenderness at the IV site

Question 289: Among the following babies, who is least likely to experience insensible water loss?

A) a 30-week-old baby in a closed Isolette incubator

B) a 28-week-old baby in an open-bed warmer

C) a 36-week-old baby in an open bassinet with a respiratory rate of 64/min

Question 290: A newborn baby named Liam is currently in the Neonatal Intensive Care Unit (NICU) and is undergoing treatment for gram-negative sepsis. He has been administered a relatively high dosage of gentamicin and ampicillin for the past three days. Apart from the potential risk of kidney damage due to the medication, what other risk is Liam exposed to?

A) Enhanced cognitive development

B) Increased risk of developing allergies

C) Hearing loss

Question 291: What adaptive response takes place when a newborn, who is on intravenous fluids, experiences hyponatremia and third spacing?

A) The neonate develops hypernatremia.

B) The neonate develops hypokalemia.

C) The neonate develops hypocalcemia.

Question 292: "What should be the initial approach of a nurse while instructing a parent on how to manage their infant's feeding tube?"

A) Immediately demonstrating the procedure without asking the parent's preference

B) Inquiring about the parent's preferred learning method

C) Telling the parent to follow the written instructions only

Question 293: Which medication would be the preferred option for managing apnea in a prematurely born infant?

A) Caffeine

B) Ibuprofen

C) Paracetamol

Question 294: What is the implication when a disease is classified as autosomal dominant?

A) The disease can only be passed on by the mother.

B) Both parents need to pass on the gene for the disease to occur.

C) One parent should pass on the gene for the disease to manifest.

Question 295: In which of the following situations is a newborn baby more prone to developing Transient Tachypnea (TTN)?
A) Babies born to mothers with gestational diabetes
B) Babies delivered by Cesarean section
C) Babies born at full term with no complications

Question 296: "What is a suitable course of action for a neonate, who has been exposed to drugs, and is having difficulty sleeping?"
A) Minimize exposure to external stimuli.
B) Increase the temperature of the neonate's room
C) Administer additional doses of drugs

Question 297: "Among the various tocolytics available, which one is generally known to have the minimal impact on the heart rate of a fetus?"
A) Indomethacin
B) Nifedipine
C) Magnesium Sulfate

Question 298: Can you describe what a patent ductus arteriosus refers to in medical terms?
A) An opening between the pulmonary and aortic arteries
B) A closure of the ductus arteriosus
C) An inflammation of the ductus arteriosus

Question 299: A newborn baby is showing mild breathing difficulties and paleness. However, on the seventh day, there is a sudden rise in pressure in the upper limbs and a drop in the lower limbs. The oxygen saturation in the right foot is 4% less than in the right hand. What medical condition could these symptoms suggest?
A) Aortic Coarctation
B) Pneumonia
C) Congenital heart disease

Question 300: In newborn babies, what is the primary cause of disseminated intravascular coagulopathy (DIC)?
A) Sepsis
B) Hypoglycemia
C) Congenital heart disease

Question 301: In the event that a newborn baby, exhibiting characteristics of Potter facies such as epicanthal folds, low-set ears, a smooth philtrum, retrognathia, and widely spaced eyes, is brought into the neonatal intensive care unit, what condition should the nurse be vigilant for in their assessment?
A) Pulmonary hypoplasia

B) Congenital heart disease
C) Down syndrome

Question 302: "Does Turner's syndrome predominantly occur in newborn boys or girls?"
A) It affects males only.
B) It affects both males and females equally.
C) It affects females newborns only.

Question 303: "What is the medical crisis that could potentially result in hypovolemic shock in a newborn?"
A) Subgalealhemorrhage
B) Mild dehydration
C) Common cold

Question 304: What potential risk could be escalated if the arm(s) of a fetus, let's say baby Thomas, becomes entwined around his head during a breech birth?
A) Meconium aspiration syndrome
B) Hyperglycemia
C) Brachial plexus injury

Question 305: What is the approximate percentage of total body water in a full-term newborn?
A) 50%
B) 90%
C) 70%

Question 306: What is the medical term for the condition that inhibits a newborn's ability to breathe immediately after birth?
A) Neonatal asphyxia
B) Bilateral choanal atresia
C) Neonatal jaundice

Question 307: A first-time mom is spending time with her newborn in the Neonatal Intensive Care Unit. She is worried about the small white spots appearing on her baby's nose and chin. How should the nurse address her concerns?
A) This is a sign of a severe skin infection and immediate medical intervention is required.
B) This is a normal part of newborn development and there is nothing to worry about.
C)This condition is a result of clogged skin pores and will naturally resolve without intervention.

Question 308: "When is the procedure of gut priming typically carried out following a baby's birth?"
A) Immediately after birth
B) 1st week of life
C) 3rd day of life

Question 309: How do the levels of an intravenous drug in a newborn baby compare to those in an adult or an older child?

A) Drug levels and the minimum effective concentration are the same in newborns and adults

B) Drug concentrations persist above the minimal effective threshold for an extended duration.

C) Drug levels drop below the minimum effective concentration faster

Question 310: What term would you use to describe a scenario in a research study where the same tool yields consistent measurements over a certain period of time?

A) Generalizability

B) Reliability

C) Validity

Question 311: A newborn baby, who has been diagnosed with a congenital diaphragmatic hernia, is experiencing intense breathing difficulties and uneven breathing sounds. What should be included in the immediate medical response?

A) Administering intravenous fluids and oxygen therapy only

B) Immediate surgical intervention without any preoperative stabilization

C) Performing intubation and implanting an orogastric tube for low intermittent suction.

Question 312: What should be the oxygen saturation level of a newborn baby, like little Emma, one minute after she is born?

A) 80% to 85%

B) 60% to 64%

C) 70% to 75%

Question 313: Which medication should not be administered to infants under two months of age due to the risk of developing kernicterus?

A) Acetaminophen

B) Sulfonamides

C) Ibuprofen

Question 314: A newborn baby is severely sick and survival chances are slim. The baby's mother, let's call her Mrs. Smith, is showing signs of emotional withdrawal and is avoiding any physical contact with the baby. What could this behavior likely indicate?

A) Mrs. Smith is experiencing anticipatory grief

B) Mrs. Smith does not feel any emotional attachment to the baby

C) Mrs. Smith is showing signs of postpartum depression

Question 315: "Which of the following is most commonly linked to the occurrence of subgaleal hemorrhages?"

A) Forceps-/vacuum-assisted delivery

B) Cesarean section

C) Spontaneous vaginal delivery

Question 316: "In the context of oxygen administration, which situation would justify the use of a nasal cannula for a baby?

A) A 28-week-old infant who is on tube-feeding and requires 0.2lpm O2 to maintain a SpO2 greater than 85%

B) An infant of 34 weeks, bottle-feeding, necessitates a 0.5 lpm O2 supply to keep SpO2 above 90%

C) A full-term infant who is breastfeeding and requires 1lpm O2 to maintain a SpO2 greater than 95%

Question 317: How would you compare the absorption of medications through the skin in preterm babies to that of full-term babies?

A) Less than in term neonates

B) Higher than in term neonates

C) The same as in term neonates

Question 318: 'For maintaining the acid-base equilibrium in a newborn's nutrition, which mineral is crucial?

A) Sodium

B) Potassium

C) Iron

Question 319: "What is the primary objective of conducting Critical Congenital Heart Disease (CCHD) tests on newborns?"

A) To detect neonates with critical congenital heart disease

B) To check the newborn's hearing ability

C) To determine the infant's blood type

Question 320: In a newborn baby experiencing shock, which condition is typically observed alongside low blood pressure and reduced blood flow?

A) Metabolic acidosis

B) Hyperglycemia

C) Polycythemia

Question 321: "What type of gastrointestinal condition could potentially develop due to malrotation?"

A) Peptic ulcer disease

B) Gastroesophageal reflux disease

C) Volvulus

Question 322: When a nurse observes a slight bluish discoloration around the mouth of a newborn, what should be the initial course of action?

A) Leave the baby alone as the bluish discoloration is a normal occurrence in newborns.

B) Immediately feed the baby to distract them from the discomfort.

C) Examine the newborn's entire body for peripheral cyanosis and observe for any retractions or indicators of respiratory distress.

Question 323: A baby named Lily is currently in the Neonatal Intensive Care Unit (NICU) receiving treatment for meningitis. The prescribed medication is ampicillin, with a dosage of 400 mg/kg/day, divided into three equal parts for every 8 hours. Lily's weight is 6 pounds and 8 ounces. Can you calculate the number of milligrams to be administered for each dose?

A) 393 mg

B) 450 mg

C) 350 mg

Question 324: What could be a potential outcome if coarctation of the aorta is not addressed in a timely manner?

A) Congestive heart failure

B) Development of extra limbs

C) Accelerated growth rate

Question 325: What should be the subsequent course of action if a newborn's heart rate drops to 40, even after receiving positive-pressure ventilation and chest compressions, two minutes post-birth?

A) Administer a glucose solution

B) Continue with chest compressions and positive-pressure ventilation

C) Administer epinephrine

Question 326: A newborn baby is being assessed by a nurse. The baby is exhibiting signs of respiratory distress, such as retracting with each breath and making a low grunting noise due to rapid breathing. What could be the most probable diagnosis for these symptoms?

A) Meconium aspiration syndrome

B) Cystic Fibrosis

C) Congenital heart disease

Question 327: "In newborns, which infection is most frequently observed?"

A) Streptococcus pneumoniae

B) Enterovirus

C) Staphylococcus aureus

Question 328: Can you explain the distinction between hypoxia and hypoxemia?

A) Hypoxia is a decrease in the oxygen level within arterial blood, while hypoxemia is decreased oxygen available at the tissue level.

B) Hypoxia and hypoxemia both refer to the same condition of decreased oxygen level in the blood.

C) Hypoxia refers to the reduced availability of oxygen at the tissue level, whereas hypoxemia denotes a lowered level of oxygen in arterial blood.

Question 329: While providing a blood transfusion to an anemic premature baby, what symptom might indicate a potential transfusion reaction?

A) Decreased heart rate

B) Tenderness at the IV site

C) Increased appetite

Question 330: In the context of transfusing blood or blood products, which of the given assertions holds true?

A) A patient with B+ blood can donate blood to a recipient of any blood type.

B) A patient with O-blood can receive blood from a donor of any blood type.

C) A patient with AB+ blood can accept blood from a donor of any blood type.

Question 331: "What is the primary course of action for managing a case of transposition of the great arteries?"

A) Administration of Diuretics

B) Immediate surgical correction without any medical intervention

C) Prostaglandin E1

Question 332: Which of the following symptoms would suggest that a patient, let's say Michael, is suffering from paralysis of both vocal cords?

A) Inspiratory stridor

B) High-pitched voice

C) Persistent coughing

Question 333: What is the primary reason for unclear genitalia in a genetically female newborn?

A) Congenital adrenal hyperplasia

B) Inadequate prenatal care

C) Maternal drug use during pregnancy

Question 334: "What is the primary immediate risk for newborns whose mothers have consumed cocaine during their gestation period?"

A) Enhanced cognitive development

B) Premature delivery

C) Increased birth weight

Question 335: Which of the following symptoms would suggest a mild case of birth asphyxia?

A) Neonate exhibiting excessive alertness for a duration of 45 to 60 minutes post-birth and possessing dilated pupils.

B) Neonate sleeping excessively and having constricted pupils

C) Neonate showing no interest in feeding and having a normal heart rate

Question 336: What is the accurate observation to make when evaluating the respiratory condition of a newborn using the Silverman-Anderson index during inhalation?

A) The abdomen and chest should rise together.

B) The abdomen should rise while the chest remains still.

C) The chest should rise while the abdomen remains still.

Question 337: "What action has been observed to reduce the occurrence of apnea in newborn babies?"

A) Rocking movement

B) Feeding the baby more frequently

C) Increasing the room temperature

Question 338: If a neonatal intensive care nurse is evaluating a newborn baby, named Lily, who has been diagnosed with tracheomalacia, what kind of observation might she potentially make during the examination?

A) Expiratory stridor

B) Cyanosis during feeding

C) Excessive drooling

Question 339: What is the minimum fill volume required to operate an automated peritoneal dialysis machine for a neonate suffering from renal failure?

A) 150 mL

B) 50 mL

C) 100 mL

Question 340: The parents of a newborn baby, diagnosed with Down syndrome, express their desire to expand their family to the nurse. However, they are worried about the potential of their future children also having this syndrome. What would be the most suitable reply to their concerns?

A) Every child they have will definitely have Down syndrome.

B) The chance of that happening is very high, about 1 out of 2 pregnancies.

C) The likelihood of that occurring is very low, approximately 1 out of 100 pregnancies.

Question 341: "What chronic condition is frequently associated with Periventricular leukomalacia?"

A) Diabetes

B) Cerebral palsy

C) Asthma

Question 342: What condition is more frequently associated with early-onset neonatal sepsis compared to late-onset neonatal sepsis?

A) Pneumonia

B) Urinary Tract Infections

C) Meningitis

Question 343: "In the context of neonatal care, which group is most frequently associated with medication errors?"

A) Infants with normal birth weight

B) Full-term infants

C) Preterm infants

Question 344: "What potential health risk does a newborn baby, infected with cytomegalovirus (CMV), face?"

A) Increased risk of developing diabetes

B) Hearing loss

C) Enhanced physical growth

Question 345: What is the usual course of treatment for a newborn, who has experienced birth asphyxia and is showing symptoms of Syndrome of Inappropriate Antidiuretic Hormone Secretion (SIADH)?

A) Administration of high doses of antibiotics

B) Fluid restriction

C) Immediate surgical intervention

Question 346: 'For what primary purpose is venovenous ECMO typically utilized?

A) To treat skin infections

B) Respiratory support

C) To increase blood pressure

Question 347: "What is the common name for the genetic condition known as trisomy 18?"

A) Down syndrome

B) Edwards syndrome

C) Turner syndrome

Question 348: "In a newborn baby's adaptive immune response, which element plays a crucial role?"

A) Platelets

B) Red blood cells

C) T-cells

Question 349: "What is the activity that has been observed to reduce the occurrence of apnea in newborn babies?"

A) Continuous Positive Airway Pressure (CPAP)

B) Rocking movement

C) Intravenous medication administration

Question 350: When it comes to the transfusion of blood or blood products, which statement holds true?

A) A patient with O- blood can receive blood from a donor of any blood type.

B) A patient with AB+ blood can accept blood from a donor of any blood type.

C) A patient with B+ blood can donate blood to a recipient of any blood type.

Question 351: "Among the listed congenital heart conditions, which one is not associated with cyanosis?"

A) Tetralogy of Fallot

B) Transposition of the great arteries

C) Ventricular septal defect

Question 352: In the case of a late-onset group B streptococcal infection, at what time frame do the symptoms usually start to manifest?

A) Between 1 week and 3 months

B) Within the first 24 hours of birth

C) After 6 months of age

Question 353: By the third day, what should be the minimum urinary output of a newborn baby?

A) 0.5 to 1 mL/kg/hr

B) 1 to 3 mL/kg/hr

C) 4 to 6 mL/kg/hr

Question 354: In the context of a child patient in the Neonatal Intensive Care Unit who has been administered a dopamine infusion, how long would it typically take for the impacts of this medication to dissipate?

A) Within 1 hour

B) Within 30 minutes

C) Within 10 minutes

Question 355: What is the suggested volume for administering normal saline as a volume expander during the resuscitation of a newborn?

A) 15 mL/kg

B) 5 mL/kg

C) 10 mL/kg

Question 356: In the case of neonatal small left colon syndrome, when do symptoms typically start to show?

A) Immediately after birth

B) After 1 week of birth

C) 24 to 36 hours of birth

Question 357: What should be the subsequent course of action if an imperforate anus is identified during the first postnatal examination of a newborn?

A) Immediately start oral feeding

B) Discharge the baby without any intervention

C) Evaluate for the presence of a fistula.

Question 358: What genetic disorder is often associated with the presence of an atrioventricular septal defect, or in milder cases, a ventricular septal defect, as observed by a Neonatal Intensive Care Unit nurse?

A) Turner syndrome

B) Marfan syndrome

C) Down syndrome

Question 359: What is the crucial step to avoid the aspiration of saliva in a newborn, named Lily, who has an intestinal obstruction and has been fitted with an NG tube?

A) That the aspirate be drained into a container and left for a few hours before being aspirated

B) That the aspirate be left to drain naturally without any intervention

C) That the aspirate drains into a drainage bag and the stomach contents be aspirated at least every 30 minutes

Question 360: "What is the primary reason for respiratory distress syndrome in a newborn baby?"

A) Neonatal sepsis

B) Newborn's Transient tachypnea

C) Congenital heart disease

Question 361: "What is the medical crisis that may result in hypovolemic shock in a newborn baby?"

A) Subgaleal hemorrhage

B) Common Cold

C) Mild Jaundice

Question 362: A 30-week pregnant woman, experiencing symptoms such as discomfort in the right upper quadrant, feelings of nausea, episodes of vomiting and high blood pressure, is most likely to be diagnosed with what condition?

A) Preeclampsia

B) Gestational Diabetes

C) HELLP syndrome

Question 363: "In newborns, hyperbilirubinemia typically leads to a rise in which specific type of bilirubin?"

A) Biliverdin

B) Unconjugated (indirect) bilirubin

C) Conjugated (direct) bilirubin

Question 364: "Which medication from the list below is not recommended for treating an infant, say baby James, who is experiencing respiratory distress?"

A) Oxygen Therapy

B) Surfactant Replacement Therapy

C) Formoterol (Perforomist)

Question 365: In the Neonatal Intensive Care Unit, a young patient is being administered a dopamine infusion. After the completion of this treatment, when should the impact of the drug be expected to dissipate?
A) Within 24 hours
B) Within 10 minutes
C) After 48 hours

Question 366: What does it suggest when a newborn, with an umbilical artery catheter inserted, shows signs of blue discoloration in their feet, also known as "catheter toes"?
A) Infection in the umbilical cord
B) Vasospasm
C) Normal reaction to the catheter

Question 367: What particular health risk are newborns suffering from short bowel syndrome and receiving parenteral nutrition particularly susceptible to?
A) Heart disease
B) Kidney stones
C) Liver failure

Question 368: What should be the optimal skin temperature range for premature babies?
A) 37 °C to 37.5 °C
B) 34.5 °C to 35 °C
C) 36 °C to 36.5 °C

Question 369: "What is typically the preferred method of treatment for a staphylococcal infection in newborns?"
A) Ibuprofen
B) Methicillin
C) Penicillin

Question 370: In a scenario where a nurse mistakenly gives an incorrect amount of medicine to a baby in the Neonatal Intensive Care Unit, leading to unfavorable results, what would this situation be termed as?
A) Medical misdiagnosis
B) Medical malpractice
C) Medical negligence

Question 371: When utilizing music therapy for a premature baby, what is the suggested volume level?
A) 100 to 110 dB
B) 65 to 75 dB
C) 85 to 95 dB

Question 372: "What is the accurate statement regarding human donor breast milk?"

A) Human donor milk is typically purchased in a grocery store.
B) Human donor milk is provided by a milk bank.
C) Human donor milk is always provided by the infant's biological mother.

Question 373: What is the typical range for maintaining positive end-expiratory pressure (PEEP) in an intubated and ventilated newborn?
A) 1 to 3 cmH2O
B) 8 to 10 cmH2O
C) 4 to 7 cmH2O

Question 374: What is the standard range for direct bilirubin in a newborn baby?
A) <<0.6 mg/dL (<<10 µmol/L)
B) 2.5 mg/dL (43 µmol/L)
C) 1.2 mg/dL (20 µmol/L)

Question 375: When it comes to continuous enteral feedings, what is the recommended duration for which breast milk or formula should be prepared and hung at once?
A) 2 hours
B) 4 hours
C) 6 hours

Question 376: A neonatal intensive care nurse has obtained a laboratory analysis of the cerebrospinal fluid (CSF) from a newborn baby named Lily, who recently had a lumbar puncture procedure. The report indicates that Lily's CSF glucose level is 100 mg/dL. What is the interpretation of this glucose level?
A) The neonate has a low CSF glucose level.
B) The neonate has a normal CSF glucose level.
C) The neonate has a high CSF glucose level.

Question 377: What does it signify if there's no visible fluctuation in the chest tube or the bottle of a newborn baby, named Lily, who has a chest tube inserted due to pneumothorax?
A) Lily's condition is improving
B) Obstruction in the chest tube
C) The chest tube is functioning properly

Question 378: What is one of the requirements for a newborn to be eligible for extracorporeal membrane oxygenation (ECMO)?
A) Weight >2,000 g
B) Weight <1,500 g
C) Newborn is older than 1 month

Question 379: What is the most effective breastfeeding position for a newborn who has a small jaw (micrognathi A) and struggles with feeding but does not have any breathing issues?

A) Laid-back position with the baby lying flat on the mother's chest

B) Cradle hold with the baby's head resting on the mother's elbow

C) Tummy to tummy with the mother reclining

Question 380: "What is typically the first surgical procedure performed on a newborn, let's say baby Jane, who is diagnosed with persistent cloaca?"

A) Tracheostomy

B) Colostomy

C) Appendectomy

Question 381: In the initial months after birth, which type of proteins is a newborn capable of digesting?

A) Red meat proteins

B) Vegetable proteins

C)Infant formula or breast milk

Question 382: What is a beneficial activity that can assist a premature baby in the Neonatal Intensive Care Unit, who is currently on tube feedings, in making the switch to oral feedings?

A) Administer a pacifier for the infant to suck during the tube feedings

B) Increase the frequency of tube feedings

C) Limit the baby's movement during feedings

Question 383: In the case of pulmonary atresia, through what means does the blood circulate to the lungs?

A) Ductus arteriosus

B) Pulmonary vein

C) Aorta

Question 384: What could be a frequent reason for a cardiac tamponade occurring in a newborn?

A) Congenital heart defects

B) Overhydration from intravenous fluids

C) Incorrect location of a central venous catheter tip

Question 385: "What is the preterm birth weight that is most commonly linked with the highest insensible water loss (IWL)?"

A) <<1,250 g

B) 1,500 g

C) 2,000 g

Question 386: What volume of medication should be administered to a newborn if they are prescribed a dose of 0.9 mg and the available concentration of the drug is 1.5 mg per 1 mL?

A) 0.6 mL

B) 0.9 mL

C) 1.2 mL

Question 387: In the scenario where a newborn baby, let's call him Baby Michael, is diagnosed with anemia and showing symptoms of hypoxemia, what would be the appropriate volume of packed red blood cells to administer in a single transfusion?

A) 10 mL/kg

B) 15 mL/kg

C) 5 mL/kg

Question 388: "What is the most frequently occurring issue associated with the use of ECMO (Extra Corporeal Membrane Oxygenation)?"

A) Hypothermia

B) Bleeding

C) Overhydration

Question 389: What hormone is released in higher amounts when a mother's nipples are stimulated?

A) Prolactin

B) Estrogen

C) Progesterone

Question 390: A newborn baby, who we'll call Lily, presents with certain facial features such as small eyes, an unusually thin upper lip, lack of a philtrum (the vertical indentation between the nose and mouth), and a smaller than average head size. What condition do these head and facial characteristics typically indicate?

A) Down Syndrome

B) Cerebral Palsy

C) Fetal alcohol syndrome

Question 391: "What is the potential outcome for infants in the Neonatal Intensive Care Unit (NICU) when a cycled lighting system (bright in the daytime and dim at night) is implemented?"

A) Infants experiencing higher rates of infection

B) Infants being able to feed sooner

C) Infants having longer hospital stays

Question 392: "What could be a frequent reason for a cardiac tamponade occurring in a newborn baby?"

A) Inadequate breastfeeding

B) Exposure to cold temperature

C)Improper positioning of the central venous catheter tip

Question 393: Using the 7-8-9-10 rule as a guideline, what would be the estimated distance from the lips to the midpoint between the glottis and carina for an endotracheal tube in a newborn baby weighing 2 kg?

A) 10CM

B) 6CM

C) 8CM

Question 394: "What is crucial for maintaining glucose balance in a newborn's body after birth?"

A) Increased intake of proteins

B) Elevated secretion of catecholamines

C) Decreased production of insulin

Question 395: "When should a blood sample be taken from a baby in the Neonatal Intensive Care Unit who is being treated with carbamazepine (Tegretol) for seizures, in order to check the drug level?"

A) Immediately prior to administering the standard scheduled dosage.

B) Two hours after administering the drug

C) Immediately after administering the drug

Question 396: "What is the suggested method for taking care of a newborn's umbilical cord?"

A) Washing with water and allowing it to air dry

B) Covering it with a bandage or plaster

C) Applying baby powder to the umbilical cord

Question 397: What is often the cause of polycythemia associated with hyperviscosity?

A) Chronic hypoxia

B) High blood glucose levels

C) Overhydration

Question 398: "What is the most probable condition that early onset group B strep infection can lead to in a newborn?"

A) Migraine

B) Asthma

C) Sepsis

Question 399: What is the standard range for serum phosphorus levels in a newborn baby?

A) 10 to 15 mg/dL (3.2 to 4.8 mmol/L)

B) 2.5 to 4.5 mg/dL (0.8 to 1.4 mmol/L)

C) 4.6 to 8 mg/dL (1.5 to 2.6 mmol/L)

Question 400: What is the suggested dosage of additional iron for a preterm neonate with low birth weight?

A) 1 mg/kg/day beginning at 1 month

B) 2 mg/kg/day beginning at 2 months

C) 3 mg/kg/day beginning at 3 months

Question 401: "What is the primary reason for high blood pressure in a prematurely born infant?"

A) Renal abnormalities

B) Overhydration

C) Genetic predisposition

Question 402: The liver is responsible for the production of procoagulant factors and regulatory proteins. However, they need a specific vitamin to be operational. Can you identify which vitamin is it?

A) Vitamin B12

B) Vitamin K

C) Vitamin C

Question 403: "What kind of diuretic has the potential to elevate the levels of calcium in the serum?"

A) Loop diuretics (furosemide)

B) Potassium-sparing diuretics (spironolactone)

C) Thiazide diuretics (hydrochlorothiazide)

Question 404: What crucial information should caregivers comprehend when a nurse is providing instructions on home-based tracheostomy care?

A) The trach tube must be replaced with a new one every time it is removed.

B) The trach tube can be reused after it has been appropriately cleaned

C) The trach tube does not need to be cleaned or maintained.

Question 405: "What could be the medical implication if a newborn baby, let's say baby Jack, shows signs of jitteriness in his limbs?"

A) Congenital Heart Disease

B) Hypocalcemia

C) Bronchopulmonary Dysplasia

Question 406: "What could be the probable cause of an early onset group B strep infection in a newborn baby?"

A) Genetic abnormalities

B) Exposure to unclean surfaces

C) Sepsis

Question 407: "What is the primary reason for infants experiencing hearing impairment?"

A) Exposure to loud noises

B)Primary cytomegalovirus infection at birth

C) Lack of prenatal vitamins during pregnancy

Question 408: What might be the suitable intervention for a newborn baby, who has a feeding tube and is experiencing vomiting, but shows no signs of any physical issues?

A) Reducing the amount of feed administered

B) Increasing the feeding volume

C) Administering antibiotics without a doctor's prescription

Question 409: In a scenario where a newborn's health is severely compromised, and the doctor informs the parents that continued treatment might only extend the baby's discomfort. Consequently, the parents decide to opt for palliative care only. Which ethical principle is being applied in this situation?

A) Autonomy

B) Nonmaleficence

C) Beneficence

Question 410: What are the signs that suggest a baby might be experiencing an excess of fluids in their system?

A) Hypertension

B) Hypotension

C) Hyperthermia

Question 411: In the initial months after birth, which type of proteins is a newborn capable of digesting?

A) Infant formula or breast milk

B) Animal-based proteins

C) Plant-based proteins

Question 412: If a novice parent, cradling a newborn who is nodding their head, clenching their hands, and smacking their lips, what should the nurse inform the parent these behaviors are indicative of?

A) Indicative of sleepiness

B) Hunger

C) Indicative of discomfort

Question 413: In which scenario would both environmental and genetic influences have an equal contribution to the occurrence of cleft lip and palate?

A) The neonate has only cleft lip and palate

B) The neonate has a cardiac defect

C) The neonate has Down Syndrome

Question 414: 'What facial expression signifies physical discomfort and suffering in a newborn baby?'

A) Yawning frequently

B) Brow bulge with vertical furrows

C) Smiling with eyes closed

Question 415: Can you explain the distinction between the assessments of total bilirubin and direct bilirubin?

A) Total bilirubin encompasses both direct and indirect bilirubin, whereas direct bilirubin refers to the unconjugated portion that typically transits from the liver to the small intestine.

B) Direct bilirubin is the total amount of bilirubin in the blood, while total bilirubin is the amount that is bound and unbound in the liver.

C) Total bilirubin refers to the amount of bilirubin excreted by the kidneys, while direct bilirubin refers to the amount absorbed by the intestines.

Question 416: A neonatal intensive care nurse is evaluating a baby boy, named Ethan, who has been diagnosed with kidney disease. In the last four hours, Ethan has produced 100 mL of urine. His weight is recorded as 6 lbs., which is approximately 2.73 kg. What would be the preliminary understanding of this situation?

A) Ethan is experiencing dehydration

B) Ethan has normal urine output

C) Ethan is experiencing severe polyuria

Question 417: What could be the possible medical indication for a newborn, if the test results show a high level of conjugated (direct) bilirubin in their blood serum?

A) Neonatal diabetes

B) Biliary atresia

C) Congenital hypothyroidism

Question 418: A newborn baby, with pink upper body and head but blue-colored legs and toes, is brought in. The baby's breathing rate is 55 breaths per minute and the heart rate is 120 beats per minute, accompanied by a noticeable murmur. What type of cyanosis is most likely being displayed in this case?

A) Central cyanosis

B) Differential cyanosis

C) Peripheral cyanosis

Question 419: In the event of metabolic alkalosis and a rise in HCO3-, what would be the compensatory process?

A) Decreased PaCO2

B) Increased PaCO2

C) No change in PaCO2

ANSWERS WITH DETAILED EXPLANATION

Answers With Detailed Explanation

Question 1:

Correct Answer: C) Tetralogy of Fallot

Explanation: Tetralogy of Fallot is a congenital heart defect characterized by four abnormalities in the heart's structure. In this condition, the newborn baby experiences severe blueness immediately after birth, known as cyanosis. This blueness occurs due to decreased blood flow to the lungs and a mixture of oxygen-rich and oxygen-poor blood. The baby also faces difficulties in feeding or crying, which further intensifies the blueness. These symptoms, specifically the blueness and feeding difficulties, strongly suggest Tetralogy of Fallot. It is essential to diagnose this condition promptly to ensure appropriate medical intervention and management for the newborn's well-being.

Question 2:

Correct Answer: C) Hypertension after 20 weeks without proteinuria

Explanation: Gestational hypertension is characterized by hypertension after 20 weeks of pregnancy without the presence of proteinuria. This condition is defined by elevated blood pressure levels, typically above 140/90 mmHg, in pregnant women who previously had normal blood pressure readings. The absence of proteinuria distinguishes gestational hypertension from preeclampsia, another hypertensive disorder of pregnancy. While preeclampsia involves both hypertension and proteinuria, gestational hypertension only involves elevated blood pressure. It is crucial to monitor and manage gestational hypertension to minimize potential risks to both the mother and the developing fetus. Regular blood pressure monitoring and close medical supervision are essential to ensure the well-being of the pregnant woman and her baby.

Question 3:

Correct Answer: B) Heart rate variability

Explanation: Heart rate variability (HRV) can be utilized as a method to evaluate the autonomic function in a newborn baby. HRV refers to the variation in time intervals between consecutive heartbeats, which is influenced by the autonomic nervous system (ANS). The ANS plays a critical role in regulating various physiological processes, including heart rate. By examining HRV, we can gain insights into the functioning of the ANS and its balance between sympathetic and parasympathetic activity. In newborns, HRV can provide valuable information about their overall health, stress levels, and resilience to various environmental challenges. Therefore, HRV analysis serves as a non-invasive and objective tool to assess autonomic function in newborn babies, aiding in early detection and management of potential health issues.

Question 4:

Correct Answer: C) Left ventrical Hypoplastic left heart syndrome (HLHS)

Explanation: Hypoplastic left heart syndrome is a heart disorder characterized by underdevelopment of the left side of the heart, including the left ventricle, aorta, and mitral valve. This condition can lead to weak pulses in the extremities and a decrease in temperature of the limbs. The underdeveloped left side of the heart affects the heart's ability to pump blood effectively, resulting in reduced blood flow to the extremities. As a result, the pulses in the limbs become weaker, and the temperature of the limbs may decrease due to decreased blood supply. It is important to recognize these symptoms as they can indicate a serious heart condition such as hypoplastic left heart syndrome.

Question 5:

Correct Answer: A) 60 to 80 mmHg

Explanation: The standard arterial blood gas (ABG) measurement for PaO2 in a newborn baby is 60 to 80 mmHg. This range is considered normal and optimal for newborns. PaO2, which stands for partial pressure of oxygen, reflects the amount of oxygen dissolved in the arterial blood. Maintaining a PaO2 level within this range is crucial for ensuring adequate oxygenation of the newborn's tissues and organs. Values below 60 mmHg may indicate hypoxemia, a condition characterized by low oxygen levels in the blood, which can lead to various complications. On the other hand, values above 80 mmHg may suggest hyperoxemia, excessive oxygen levels in the blood, which can also be harmful. Therefore, a PaO2 measurement of 60 to 80 mmHg is considered the standard and desirable range for newborn babies.

Question 6:

Correct Answer: C) >150 mg/dL

Explanation: A hyperglycemic condition in a premature newborn is characterized by blood glucose levels above 150 mg/dL. This elevated blood glucose level indicates a state of hyperglycemia, which can have detrimental effects on the infant's health. High blood glucose levels in premature newborns can lead to various complications, such as increased risk of infection, respiratory distress, and impaired neurological development. It is crucial to closely monitor and manage blood glucose levels in premature infants to prevent these adverse outcomes. Maintaining blood glucose levels within the appropriate range is essential for promoting optimal growth, development, and overall well-being of premature newborns.

Question 7:

Correct Answer: C) Elevated likelihood of premature delivery

Explanation: A positive result on a Kleihauer-Betke test suggests an increased risk of preterm birth, especially when a mother has experienced a traumatic event like a car accident. This test is used to detect fetal-maternal hemorrhage, which is the leakage of fetal blood into the maternal circulation. In cases of trauma, such as a car accident, the uterus can experience sudden and intense pressure, leading to potential placental damage and subsequent bleeding. This fetal-maternal hemorrhage can result in the loss of fetal red blood cells into the maternal bloodstream. A positive Kleihauer-Betke test indicates the presence of these fetal red blood cells, indicating a higher likelihood of preterm birth. Monitoring and appropriate management are crucial in such situations to ensure the well-being of both the mother and the baby.

Question 8:

Correct Answer: B) Conversation

Explanation: Conversation contributes the most to the level of noise in a Neonatal Intensive Care Unit (NICU). The constant chatter and communication between healthcare professionals, patients' families, and visitors can significantly increase noise levels in the unit. Conversations are essential for conveying information, discussing patient care, and providing emotional support. However, the noise generated from these conversations can have adverse effects on the delicate environment of the NICU. Excessive noise can disrupt the sleep patterns of newborns, increase stress levels, and potentially impact their neurodevelopment. Therefore, it is crucial for healthcare providers to be mindful of their conversations and take necessary measures to minimize noise in order to optimize the healing environment for the vulnerable infants in the NICU.

Question 9:

Correct Answer: B) The foreskin should be completely retracted for cleaning and the area should be dried well.

Explanation: The foreskin should be completely retracted for cleaning and the area should be dried well. This is an important aspect of care for uncircumcised boys, as it helps to prevent the accumulation of smegma, a substance that can build up under the foreskin and lead to infections. By retracting the foreskin and ensuring that the area is thoroughly cleaned and dried, parents can maintain good hygiene and reduce the risk of complications. It is important to note that this should be done gently and without force, as the foreskin may still be attached to the glans in newborns. Regularly incorporating this practice into their care guidelines will help parents ensure the well-being and comfort of their uncircumcised baby boy.

Question 10:

Correct Answer: C) Phenytoin (Dilantin) with D5W

Explanation: Phenytoin (Dilantin) with D5W is a safe combination of medications that can be administered together via an intravenous route. Phenytoin is an anticonvulsant medication used to treat seizures, while D5W is a type of intravenous solution that provides dextrose and water. When these two medications are combined, they do not interact or interfere with each other's efficacy. Phenytoin helps control seizures, while D5W provides necessary fluids and nutrients to the body. This combination is commonly used in clinical settings to ensure the safe and effective administration of phenytoin while maintaining hydration. It is important to note that medication combinations should always be prescribed and administered by a qualified healthcare professional to ensure patient safety and optimal therapeutic outcomes.

Question 11:

Correct Answer: B) Stimulating the infant

Explanation: Stimulating the infant is an example of the didactic caregiving pattern. Didactic caregiving refers to a parenting style that focuses on actively teaching and guiding the child's development. By engaging in activities that stimulate the infant, such as providing age-appropriate toys, playing games that encourage exploration and learning, and encouraging sensory experiences, parents can create a stimulating environment that promotes the child's cognitive, physical, and emotional development. Through these interactions, the infant receives valuable opportunities to learn and grow, developing important skills and abilities. This approach to caregiving helps to foster a strong foundation for the child's overall development and sets the stage for future learning and exploration.

Question 12:

Correct Answer: B) Infant at 34 weeks, with a weight of 2400 g, having a respiratory rate of 42/min, placed in an oxyhood on 30% FiO2.

Explanation: In the case of a 34-week-old infant weighing 2400 g, with a respiratory rate of 42/min, and receiving oxygen therapy through an oxyhood at FiO230%, mechanical ventilation is not necessary. Mechanical ventilation is typically employed when a patient's respiratory function is severely compromised and they are unable to maintain adequate oxygenation and ventilation on their own. However, in this particular situation, the infant's respiratory rate is within the normal range, and the use of an oxyhood with a low FiO2 suggests that their oxygenation needs are being met. Therefore, the patient does not require the use of mechanical ventilation.

Question 13:

Correct Answer: C) 60 minutes

Explanation: The recommended duration for the infusion of IV ganciclovir in a newborn diagnosed with congenital cytomegalovirus infection is 60 minutes. This specific duration is crucial as it ensures optimal drug delivery and minimizes the risk of adverse reactions. By administering the infusion over 60 minutes, the medication can be properly metabolized and distributed throughout the newborn's system, effectively targeting the cytomegalovirus infection. This duration allows for a controlled and steady release of the medication, maximizing its therapeutic effects while minimizing the potential for toxicity. Therefore, it is essential to adhere to the recommended 60-minute infusion duration to ensure the safe and effective treatment of congenital cytomegalovirus infection in newborns.

Question 14:

Correct Answer: A) Oligohydramnios

Explanation: Oligohydramnios is a condition characterized by a decreased amount of amniotic fluid surrounding the fetus in the womb. When a near-term fetus, such as Baby Anthony, generates between 200 to 400 mL of urine each day, it suggests a reduced production of amniotic fluid. This can lead to complications as the amniotic fluid plays a crucial role in the development and protection of the fetus. Insufficient amniotic fluid can result in restricted fetal movement, abnormal fetal positioning, and poor lung development. It can also indicate potential issues with fetal kidney function or placental insufficiency. Therefore, it is essential to monitor amniotic fluid levels closely and consult with a medical professional to determine the underlying cause and appropriate management for Baby Anthony.

Question 15:

Correct Answer: A) >160 bpm for â‰¥10 minutes

Explanation: Tachycardia refers to an abnormally high heart rate, and it is crucial to monitor the fetal heart rate during labor to ensure the well-being of the baby. In this context, a fetal heart rate would be categorized as experiencing tachycardia when it exceeds 160 beats per minute (bpm) for a duration of at least 10 minutes. This threshold is used as a guideline to identify potential issues that may arise during labor. It is important to promptly recognize and address tachycardia as it can be an indication of fetal distress or underlying complications. By closely monitoring the fetal heart rate and identifying tachycardia, healthcare professionals can provide appropriate interventions and ensure the best possible outcome for both the mother and the baby.

Question 16:

Correct Answer: C) 8 to 10 inches

Explanation: The approximate distance at which a full-term newborn's eyes can focus is 8 to 10 inches. During the early stages of life, a newborn's visual system is still developing, and their ability to focus on objects is limited. The distance of 8 to 10 inches is significant because it is the typical distance between a newborn's face and their parent's face during feeding or bonding activities. At this distance, the newborn can begin to focus on the parent's face, making eye contact and establishing a connection. This proximity also allows the newborn to discern facial features and expressions, aiding in the development of social and emotional bonds. As the newborn grows and their visual system matures, their ability to focus will improve, and they will gradually be able to see objects at greater distances.

Question 17:

Correct Answer: A) 32 weeks of gestation

Explanation: At 32 weeks of gestation, it is crucial to shield the eyes of a prematurely born neonate from light. This specific gestational age is significant because the retina, which is the light-sensitive part of the eye, undergoes development during the late stages of pregnancy. Premature infants have an increased risk of developing retinopathy of prematurity (ROP), a condition where the blood vessels in the retina abnormally grow and can cause vision problems or even blindness. Exposure to bright lights, such as those found in the neonatal intensive care unit (NICU), can further exacerbate this condition. Therefore, shielding their eyes from light is essential to protect the delicate and developing retina of these premature neonates.

Question 18:

Correct Answer: B) 12 hours

Explanation: The recommended timeframe for a newborn baby, whose mother is infected with hepatitis B, to receive both the hepatitis B immune globulin and the hepatitis B vaccine is within 12 hours of birth. The administration of these preventive measures within this critical timeframe is crucial in preventing the transmission of the disease from the infected mother to the baby. By providing the hepatitis B immune globulin and vaccine soon after birth, the infant receives immediate protection against the virus and reduces the risk of developing chronic hepatitis B infection later in life. This prompt intervention ensures that the baby receives the maximum benefit from these preventive measures, safeguarding their health and well-being.

Question 19:

Correct Answer: B) Tetralogy of Fallot

Explanation: Tetralogy of Fallot is a well-known congenital heart anomaly that is recognized as a condition causing cyanosis. This condition is characterized by a combination of four specific heart defects: a ventricular septal defect (VSD), pulmonary stenosis, an overriding aorta, and right ventricular hypertrophy. The presence of these defects disrupts the normal flow of blood through the heart and lungs, leading to reduced oxygenation of the blood. As a result, the oxygen-depleted blood is pumped out to the body, causing a bluish discoloration of the skin and mucous membranes, known as cyanosis. Therefore, Tetralogy of Fallot is acknowledged as a congenital heart anomaly that causes cyanosis due to the abnormal flow of oxygenated and deoxygenated blood within the heart.

Question 20:

Correct Answer: B)Choanal atresia

Explanation: Choanal atresia is a medical condition that can prevent the use of nasal Continuous Positive Airway Pressure (CPAP). Choanal atresia is a congenital condition where there is a blockage or narrowing of the nasal passages at the back of the nose, specifically at the choanae. This obstruction hinders the flow of air through the nasal passages, making it difficult for individuals to breathe through their nose. As CPAP therapy relies on delivering a continuous stream of air through the nasal passages to maintain an open airway during sleep, the presence of choanal atresia can significantly impede the effectiveness of CPAP treatment. Therefore, individuals with choanal atresia may require alternative forms of respiratory support or surgical intervention to address the obstruction and improve their breathing.

Question 21:

Correct Answer: B) Infants being able to feed sooner

Explanation: Infants being able to feed sooner is a potential outcome when a cycled lighting system, with bright lights during the daytime and dim lights at night, is implemented in the Neonatal Intensive Care Unit (NICU). This lighting system helps regulate the circadian rhythm of the infants, mimicking a natural day-night cycle. Research suggests that maintaining a consistent light-dark pattern can improve an infant's feeding patterns by increasing their alertness during the day and promoting better sleep at night. When infants are more alert and less fatigued, they are more likely to be awake and receptive to feeding cues. Therefore, implementing a cycled lighting system in the NICU may contribute to improved feeding outcomes for these vulnerable infants.

Question 22:

Correct Answer: B)Post the second year of existence

Explanation: After the second year of life, a child diagnosed with late congenital syphilis typically begins to exhibit symptoms. Late congenital syphilis refers to the manifestation of syphilis infection that occurs after the first two years of life. This period is characterized by the onset of various symptoms, including bone deformities, joint swelling, rash, fever, and enlargement of the liver and spleen. The delayed appearance of these symptoms is due to the slow progression of the disease, which can remain dormant for several years before becoming symptomatic. Therefore, it is crucial to closely monitor children who have been diagnosed with congenital syphilis, as symptoms may not be apparent until after the second year of life.

Question 23:

Correct Answer: C) 67

Explanation: The caloric content per deciliter of colostrum is 67. Colostrum, also known as the first milk produced by mammals after giving birth, is crucial for providing essential nutrients and antibodies to newborns. Research has shown that colostrum is particularly rich in proteins, carbohydrates, fats, vitamins, and minerals, which contribute to its high caloric value. With a caloric content of 67 per deciliter, colostrum serves as a vital source of energy for the newborn, aiding in their growth and development. The precise composition of colostrum may vary among species, but its significance in providing optimal nutrition to newborns remains consistent.

Question 24:

Correct Answer: C) <45 dB

Explanation: The noise level recommended by the American Academy of Pediatrics (AAP) for a Neonatal Intensive Care Unit (NICU) is <45 dB. This guideline is based on extensive research and understanding of the delicate nature of newborns' auditory development and overall well-being. Noise levels above 45 dB can have adverse effects on premature infants, including increased stress levels, disrupted sleep patterns, and potential hearing damage. Keeping the noise level below this threshold helps create a more conducive environment for infants to thrive and heal. It is crucial for healthcare professionals and staff to strictly adhere to this recommendation to ensure optimal care and development for the vulnerable newborns in the NICU.

Question 25:

Correct Answer: A) Hearing test

Explanation: Hearing is the type of examination that parents or caregivers of a newborn, who has been treated for bacterial meningitis, should be advised to arrange for their baby within a timeframe of 4 to 6 weeks after discharge. Bacterial meningitis can have serious consequences on a child's auditory system, leading to hearing loss or other auditory impairments. Therefore, it is crucial to monitor the baby's hearing abilities to ensure early detection and intervention if any issues arise. By scheduling a hearing examination, healthcare professionals can assess the baby's auditory function, identify any potential hearing deficits, and provide appropriate interventions or referrals as needed. This examination plays a vital role in promoting the child's overall development and ensuring optimal communication and language skills.

Question 26:

Correct Answer: A) Decreased heart rate

Explanation: Cycled light in the Neonatal Intensive Care Unit (NICU) can have a significant impact on the physiological responses of premature infants. One of the impacts is the observed decrease in heart rate. The fluctuating light exposure mimics the natural variations in light intensity that babies would experience in the womb. When exposed to cycled light, premature infants exhibit a decrease in heart rate, indicating a calming effect on their autonomic nervous system. This decrease in heart rate is beneficial as it promotes a more stable and regulated cardiovascular system in these vulnerable infants. Furthermore, it can contribute to improved overall health outcomes and enhance the development of newborns in the NICU.

Question 27:

Correct Answer: A) An omphalocele refers to the protrusion of abdominal contents through the umbilicus, while in a gastroschisis, the abdominal organs lack a protective membrane covering

Explanation: An omphalocele occurs when the abdominal contents protrude through the umbilicus, but a gastroschisis occurs when there is no membrane covering the abdominal organs. In the case of an omphalocele, there is a protective sac or membrane that surrounds the protruding organs, which can vary in size. This sac is formed by the peritoneum and amnion. On the other hand, a gastroschisis is characterized by a defect in the abdominal wall, typically to the right of the umbilicus, that allows the intestines to freely protrude outside the body without any covering or sac. The absence of a protective membrane in gastroschisis makes it more prone to complications such as infection and damage to the exposed organs. Therefore, it is crucial to differentiate between these two conditions, as their management and prognosis may differ significantly.

Question 28:

Correct Answer: C) Shoulder dystocia

Explanation: Shoulder dystocia is a medical condition that a newborn, who is significantly larger than the average size for his gestational age, is more likely to be susceptible to. This condition occurs during childbirth when the baby's shoulders become impacted behind the mother's pubic bone, resulting in difficulty in delivering the shoulders. The increased size of the baby can put pressure on the birth canal, making it challenging for the shoulders to pass through. This can lead to complications such as brachial plexus injuries, fractured bones, and damage to the mother's birth canal. Identifying the risk factors, such as a larger baby, and taking appropriate measures during delivery, such as using certain maneuvers or performing a cesarean section, can help prevent or manage shoulder dystocia.

Question 29:

Correct Answer: B)) Perinatal asphyxia

Explanation: Perinatal asphyxia is the primary reason for sudden kidney damage in newborns. It occurs when there is a lack of oxygen supply to the baby's brain and vital organs during the birth process. This can lead to a cascade of events that ultimately result in kidney damage. When the baby's organs, including the kidneys, do not receive enough oxygen, they may experience ischemia (lack of blood flow) and subsequent cell death. This can impair the kidney's ability to filter waste products from the blood and maintain fluid and electrolyte balance. As a result, sudden kidney damage can occur, leading to potential long-term complications if not promptly addressed. It is crucial for healthcare professionals to identify and manage perinatal asphyxia promptly in order to prevent or minimize kidney damage in newborns.

Question 30:

Correct Answer: C) Vasodilation

Explanation: Vasodilation is the typical physiological reaction observed when a premature baby, born at 34 weeks of gestation, experiences hyperthermia. This process involves the dilation or widening of blood vessels in response to increased body temperature. Vasodilation allows for increased blood flow to the skin's surface, aiding in heat dissipation through radiation and convection. By expanding the blood vessels, more warm blood reaches the skin, promoting heat loss and helping to regulate the baby's body temperature. It is important to note that vasodilation is a natural mechanism that the body employs to maintain homeostasis and prevent overheating.

Question 31:

Correct Answer: B) Blood glucose

Explanation: Blood glucose is the initial diagnostic test that should be conducted when a newborn baby, such as baby Daniel, experiences a seizure. Seizures in newborns can be caused by various factors, including low blood glucose levels. By measuring the blood glucose level, healthcare professionals can quickly identify if low blood sugar is the cause of the seizure. This diagnostic test is essential as it helps determine the appropriate treatment and management for the baby. Other diagnostic tests may be conducted subsequently to identify the underlying cause of the low blood glucose, but blood glucose measurement is the first step in assessing and addressing the immediate concern of a seizure in a newborn.

Question 32:

Correct Answer: B)Accelerated PDA closure

Explanation: More rapid PDA closure is a well-known advantage of the kangaroo care method. This method involves skin-to-skin contact between a parent and their newborn, providing numerous benefits for both the baby and the parent. While it is important to exclude the advantage of more rapid PDA closure, there are several other well-established advantages of kangaroo care. These include improved bonding between parent and baby, enhanced breastfeeding success, better temperature regulation for the newborn, reduced stress levels for both parent and baby, improved sleep patterns, and increased weight gain in preterm infants. These benefits highlight the holistic advantages of kangaroo care, making it a highly recommended practice in neonatal care.

Question 33:

Correct Answer: C) Late-onset meningitis

Explanation: Late-onset meningitis is a condition that occurs in newborns after the first week of birth. In the case of Ethan, his symptoms of near-unconsciousness, protruding anterior fontanel, seizures, and impaired cranial nerves are indicative of this condition. Late-onset meningitis is typically caused by bacteria such as Group B Streptococcus, Escherichia coli, or Listeria monocytogenes, which can infect the baby through the bloodstream or during delivery. The infection can then spread to the meninges, the protective membranes surrounding the brain and spinal cord, leading to inflammation and a range of neurological symptoms. Prompt diagnosis and treatment with intravenous antibiotics are crucial to prevent long-term complications and ensure the baby's well-being.

Question 34:

Correct Answer: C) Hemoglobin less than 0.7 g/dL

Explanation: Hemoglobin less than 0.7 g/dL is a potential risk factor for the onset of severe enterovirus disease. Hemoglobin is a protein present in red blood cells that carries oxygen throughout the body. Low levels of hemoglobin indicate anemia, which can weaken the immune system and make individuals more susceptible to infections, including enterovirus. Severe enterovirus disease can lead to complications such as meningitis, encephalitis, and myocarditis, which can be life-threatening. Therefore, individuals with hemoglobin levels below 0.7 g/dL are at a higher risk of developing severe enterovirus disease due to their compromised immune system. It is important to identify and address low hemoglobin levels promptly to reduce the risk of severe enterovirus infections.

Question 35:

Correct Answer: A) 80% to 90%

Explanation: Breastfeeding is a crucial aspect of a baby's growth and development. At three months old, a full-term baby like Emma can achieve a significant portion of her total feeding within the initial 5 minutes of active nursing, specifically around 80% to 90%. During this time, the baby's suckling reflex is at its strongest, allowing for efficient milk transfer. The breast milk received during this period is rich in foremilk, which is higher in protein and hydrating properties. This concentrated nutrition provides Emma with essential nutrients and hydration required for healthy growth. It is important to note that breastfeeding is a dynamic process, and individual variations may occur. Regular monitoring and consultation with a healthcare professional are essential to ensure Emma's proper nourishment and well-being.

Question 36:

Correct Answer: B) Maintaining up-to-date knowledge and skills

Explanation: Keeping knowledge and skills current is an essential aspect of being a conscientious and accountable neonatal intensive care nurse. In order to provide the highest quality care to fragile newborns, nurses must stay up-to-date with the latest advancements, research, and evidence-based practices in neonatal care. This entails continuously engaging in professional development activities such as attending workshops, conferences, and seminars, as well as actively seeking out new information through literature reviews and online resources. By staying informed, nurses can ensure they are utilizing the most effective interventions and techniques to promote the health and well-being of their patients. Additionally, maintaining current knowledge and skills allows nurses to confidently adapt to changes in practice guidelines and provide safe and competent care to neonates and their families.

Question 37:

Correct Answer: B) Newborns weighing ≤1,500 g

Explanation: ≤1,500 g is the correct answer. According to the guidelines set by the American Academy of Pediatrics (AAP), it is suggested that all newborns weighing ≤1,500 g undergo eye examinations to identify any indications of retinopathy of prematurity. Retinopathy of prematurity is a potentially blinding condition that affects the blood vessels in the retina of premature infants. It is more common in babies born at very low birth weights, and those weighing ≤1,500 g are at higher risk. Early detection and intervention are crucial in preventing vision loss or blindness. Therefore, the AAP recommends eye examinations for these newborns to ensure timely diagnosis and appropriate management of retinopathy of prematurity.

Question 38:

Correct Answer: B) To infants in severe respiratory distress that did not respond to CPAP

Explanation: For infants in severe respiratory distress who did not respond to CPAP, it would be appropriate to administer surfactant. Surfactant is a substance that helps reduce surface tension in the lungs, allowing the alveoli to remain open and preventing their collapse during exhalation. This is crucial for proper gas exchange and adequate oxygenation in newborns. Despite the use of CPAP (Continuous Positive Airway Pressure), some infants may still struggle to maintain adequate respiratory function, and surfactant administration becomes necessary. By delivering exogenous surfactant directly into the lungs, the baby's respiratory distress can be alleviated, preventing further complications and promoting better oxygenation. Therefore, surfactant administration is an appropriate intervention for newborns in severe respiratory distress unresponsive to CPAP.

Question 39:

Correct Answer: A) Early to mid-childhood

Explanation: Early to mid-childhood is the typical age by which a newborn diagnosed with autosomal-recessive polycystic kidney disease (ARPK) is expected to progress to end-stage renal disease. ARPKD is a genetic disorder that affects the development of the kidneys and can lead to the formation of cysts in the kidneys. The progression to end-stage renal disease in ARPKD varies among individuals, but generally occurs within the first few years of life. The disease can cause significant damage to the kidneys, leading to a decline in renal function. Without proper medical intervention, such as kidney transplantation or dialysis, these children may develop end-stage renal disease by early to mid-childhood. Early diagnosis and management are crucial to delay the progression of the disease and improve the overall prognosis for these patients.

Question 40:

Correct Answer: C) The potential for long-term fertility implications due to this is considerably minimal.

Explanation: There is a very low chance of neonatal testicular torsion causing any fertility issues long-term. Although the loss of one testicle is unfortunate, the unaffected testicle should be able to compensate for the loss and produce sufficient levels of testosterone and sperm. The remaining testicle will undergo a compensatory increase in size and function to maintain normal hormonal balance and fertility potential. It is important to note that the loss of one testicle does not automatically result in infertility. However, it is recommended to monitor the child's development and seek regular medical check-ups to ensure optimal reproductive health in the future.

Question 41:

Correct Answer: C) 36 hours

Explanation: Transient tachypnea of the newborn (TTN) is a respiratory condition that typically manifests within 36 hours of birth. This delay in symptom onset is due to the delayed clearance of fetal lung fluid, resulting in excessive fluid accumulation in the lungs. As a result, newborns with TTN may experience rapid breathing, grunting, and retractions. It is important to note that while the signs of TTN usually appear within 36 hours, they can sometimes manifest as early as a few hours after birth or as late as 72 hours after delivery. However, the majority of cases present within the first day and a half, highlighting the significance of the 36-hour timeframe in diagnosing and managing TTN.

Question 42:

Correct Answer: B) Postpartum coagulopathy and hemorrhage

Explanation: Postpartum coagulopathy and hemorrhage are crucial conditions that need to be closely observed in a pregnant woman like Lisa who experiences abruptio placenta due to a car accident. Postpartum coagulopathy refers to the impaired blood clotting ability after childbirth, which can lead to excessive bleeding. This condition is particularly concerning for Lisa, as abruptio placenta is associated with a higher risk of blood clotting disorders. Furthermore, the trauma caused by the accident can potentially worsen the clotting abnormalities. Hemorrhage, on the other hand, is a significant risk due to the detachment of the placenta and subsequent disruption of the blood supply. Monitoring Lisa closely for signs of postpartum coagulopathy and hemorrhage is crucial for early detection and prompt management, ensuring the best possible outcome for both Lisa and her baby.

Question 43:

Correct Answer: C) 20

Explanation: The additional 2 g/kg/day of protein provided to baby Michael during total parenteral nutrition (TPN) contributes to an increased requirement for nonprotein energy kilocalories. To calculate the necessary energy intake, we can consider that every 1 g of protein yields approximately 4 kilocalories. Since baby Michael is receiving an extra 2 g/kg/day of protein, this equates to 8 kilocalories per kilogram per day. If we assume baby Michael's weight to be 2.5 kg, the total additional energy requirement would be 20 kilocalories (8 kilocalories/kg/day * 2.5 kg). Therefore, an additional 20 nonprotein energy kilocalories would be necessary to meet baby Michael's increased protein intake

Question 44:

Correct Answer: C) Heightened Mortality Risk

Explanation: Increased risk of death: A high serum lactate level in a baby being cared for in the Neonatal Intensive Care Unit (NICU) indicates a concerning physiological condition. Elevated lactate levels can be indicative of significant tissue hypoperfusion and impaired oxygen delivery, suggesting compromised organ function. This can be caused by various factors, such as sepsis, respiratory distress, or cardiac abnormalities. The high lactate level indicates a state of metabolic acidosis, which can lead to organ dysfunction and ultimately increase the risk of death in the neonate. Prompt identification and appropriate management of the underlying cause are crucial to improving outcomes for these vulnerable infants in the NICU.

Question 45:

Correct Answer: B) Retinopathy of prematurity (ROP)

Explanation: Retinopathy of prematurity (ROP) was the primary reason for childhood blindness in the United States during the mid-20th century, particularly in the 1940s and 1950s. ROP refers to an eye disorder that affects premature infants, causing abnormal blood vessel growth in the retina. This condition predominantly affected premature babies who required supplemental oxygen therapy, which was increasingly used during this time to treat respiratory distress syndrome. The high levels of oxygen administered to premature infants led to the development of abnormal blood vessels in the retina, leading to retinal detachment and subsequent blindness. ROP's prevalence during this period was a result of the medical advancements in neonatal care and the increased survival rate of premature infants.

Question 46:

Correct Answer: C) Failure to pass meconium in 48 hours

Explanation: Failure to pass meconium in 48 hours is a significant sign of Hirschsprung disease in a newborn baby. Meconium is a dark, sticky substance that accumulates in the baby's intestines during pregnancy. Normally, it is expelled within the first 24 to 48 hours after birth. However, in babies with Hirschsprung disease, there is a lack of nerve cells in certain segments of the colon, leading to an obstruction and the inability to pass meconium. This can result in a distended abdomen, vomiting, constipation, and poor feeding. Recognizing the failure to pass meconium in the first 48 hours is crucial in diagnosing Hirschsprung disease early and initiating appropriate treatment to prevent complications.

Question 47:

Correct Answer: A) Lift by the buttocks

Explanation: Lift by the buttocks is the crucial step to remember when changing the diaper of a newborn baby diagnosed with osteogenesis imperfecta. This is because babies with osteogenesis imperfecta have fragile bones that are prone to fractures. Lifting the baby by the buttocks, instead of the legs, helps to minimize the risk of accidental fractures. This technique ensures that the weight is evenly distributed and reduces the strain on their fragile bones. It is important to handle these babies with extreme caution and gentleness during diaper changes to prevent any unnecessary harm or discomfort.

Question 48:

Correct Answer: B) 50 mg

Explanation: In the given scenario, baby Noah weighs 2.5 kg and requires a medication dosage of 40 mg/kg/day, split into two doses. To calculate the medication dosage for each dose, we multiply baby Noah's weight by the prescribed dosage. So, for baby Noah, the medication dosage would be 40 mg/kg/day multiplied by 2.5 kg, which equals 100 mg/day. Since the medication needs to be split into two doses, we divide the total daily dosage by two. Therefore, each dose of medication for baby Noah would contain 50 mg. This ensures that baby Noah receives the prescribed dosage of 40 mg per kilogram of body weight, while also adhering to the requirement of splitting the medication into two doses.

Question 49:

Correct Answer: A) 0.5 (1:2)

Explanation: The appropriate ratio of cuff width to arm circumference when utilizing an oscillometric device to track a neonate's blood pressure is 0.5 (1:2). This ratio is crucial as it ensures accurate and reliable blood pressure measurements in neonates. A cuff that is too narrow or too wide can result in incorrect readings and compromise patient care. By using a cuff width that is half the circumference of the neonate's arm, we can achieve optimal compression and proper fit, allowing for accurate blood pressure measurements. This ratio of 0.5 (1:2) minimizes the risk of cuff-related errors and ensures precise monitoring of blood pressure in neonates.

Question 50:

Correct Answer: C) Conductive

Explanation: Conductive heat loss is the type of heat loss that occurs when a newborn, like baby Mia, is placed on a chilly surface. Conductive heat transfer happens when there is direct contact between two objects with different temperatures. In this case, when baby Mia is laid down on a cold surface, the heat from her body is transferred directly to the surface through conduction. This can cause her body temperature to decrease rapidly, putting her at risk of hypothermia. It is important to ensure that newborns are not exposed to cold surfaces for extended periods to prevent excessive heat loss and maintain their body temperature.

Question 51:

Correct Answer: C) To infants in severe respiratory distress who did not respond to CPAP

Explanation: To infants in severe respiratory distress that did not respond to CPAP, administration of a surfactant is warranted. Surfactant is a naturally occurring substance that helps reduce surface tension in the lungs, allowing the alveoli to remain open and preventing them from collapsing during exhalation. In newborns, surfactant deficiency is a common cause of respiratory distress syndrome (RDS), a condition characterized by difficulty breathing. While continuous positive airway pressure (CPAP) is typically the first-line treatment for RDS, some infants may not adequately respond to it. In such cases, surfactant therapy becomes necessary to improve lung function, enhance oxygenation, and prevent complications associated with severe respiratory distress. Therefore, surfactants should be considered as a therapeutic option for newborns who do not show improvement with CPAP alone.

Question 52:

Correct Answer: B) Birth to 5 days postpartum

Explanation: The passage of meconium in newborn babies with an extremely low birth weight (ELBW) typically occurs within 2 to 5 days of birth. Meconium is the first stool passed by a newborn, consisting of substances ingested during fetal life. In ELBW infants, meconium passage may be delayed due to their immature digestive system. The transitional process from intrauterine to extrauterine life takes longer in ELBW infants, leading to delayed bowel movements. This delay is considered normal for this specific population, and healthcare professionals closely monitor the baby's bowel movements to ensure that meconium passage occurs within the expected timeframe.

Question 53:

Correct Answer: B) Saliva

Explanation: Saliva is the substance typically utilized in diagnosing a newborn with a congenital cytomegalovirus (CMV) infection. This is due to the fact that CMV can be detected in saliva samples, making it a reliable diagnostic tool. Saliva testing offers several advantages, including ease of sample collection, non-invasive nature, and high sensitivity. By analyzing saliva samples, healthcare professionals can accurately detect the presence of CMV in newborns, allowing for early intervention and appropriate treatment. Saliva-based diagnostics have proven to be an effective and efficient method in diagnosing congenital CMV infections, ultimately contributing to better health outcomes for newborns.

Question 54:

Correct Answer: B) Within 1 hour of birth

Explanation: Within 1 hour of birth is the optimal period to administer surfactant for a newborn baby experiencing respiratory distress. This is because surfactant plays a crucial role in reducing surface tension in the alveoli, preventing their collapse and promoting proper lung function. Administering surfactant within the first hour allows for early intervention, ensuring that the baby receives the necessary support for their respiratory system as soon as possible. This early administration of surfactant can significantly improve outcomes and reduce the risk of complications associated with respiratory distress in newborns. Therefore, it is vital to prioritize the timely administration of surfactant within the first hour of birth for infants experiencing respiratory distress.

Question 55:

Correct Answer: B) 33 to 36 weeks of gestation

Explanation: Between 33 to 36 weeks of gestation, a baby typically develops the ability to coordinate sucking and swallowing. At this stage, the neurological and muscular systems necessary for these vital functions have matured enough to allow for efficient feeding. The sucking reflex is initiated by the baby's lips, tongue, and jaw, while the swallowing reflex allows the food to move from the mouth to the stomach. This coordination is crucial for the baby to obtain nutrition from breast milk or formula. It is important to note that premature babies may require additional support and monitoring to ensure proper development of these skills.

Question 56:

Correct Answer: B) Breakdown of red blood cells, increased hepatic enzyme levels, and a reduction in platelets

Explanation: HELLP syndrome is a serious maternal condition that is characterized by a specific set of symptoms: hemolysis, elevated liver enzymes, and low platelet count. Hemolysis refers to the breakdown of red blood cells, resulting in a reduction in their number and function. Elevated liver enzymes indicate liver damage or dysfunction, which can lead to a range of complications. Lastly, a low platelet count means that the blood's ability to clot is compromised, increasing the risk of excessive bleeding. These symptoms collectively define HELLP syndrome and are vital for its diagnosis. Recognizing and promptly treating this condition is crucial to ensure the well-being and safety of both the mother and the baby.

Question 57:

Correct Answer: B) Hypoperfusion

Explanation: Hypoperfusion is a condition characterized by inadequate blood supply to body tissues, resulting in reduced oxygen and nutrient delivery. In the case of Lily, a newborn baby suffering from congestive heart failure, a lactic acid level of 40 mg/dL (4.44 mmol/L) suggests the presence of hypoperfusion. This elevated lactic acid level indicates a state of tissue hypoxia, where insufficient oxygen is being delivered to the cells. In congestive heart failure, the heart is unable to pump blood effectively, leading to diminished cardiac output and compromised tissue perfusion. As a result, the body resorts to anaerobic metabolism, leading to the production of lactic acid. Therefore, Lily's lactic acid level serves as a marker for the impaired circulation and inadequate tissue oxygenation associated with congestive heart failure.

Question 58:

Correct Answer: A) 24 to 72 hours

Explanation: The recommended timeframe for conducting a screening test for phenylketonuria (PKU) is within 24 to 72 hours after birth. This timeframe is crucial because early detection and intervention can prevent severe complications associated with PKU. PKU is an inherited metabolic disorder that affects the body's ability to break down an amino acid called phenylalanine. If left untreated, high levels of phenylalanine can lead to intellectual disability, developmental delays, and other neurological problems. By conducting the screening test within the first few days of life, healthcare professionals can identify affected infants and initiate dietary modifications promptly. This early intervention can help individuals with PKU lead healthier lives and minimize the risk of long-term complications.

Question 59:

Correct Answer: B) Liver immaturity

Explanation: Liver immaturity is typically the primary reason for direct hyperbilirubinemia in a newborn baby. During the early stages of life, a baby's liver is still developing and may not be fully equipped to handle the breakdown and elimination of bilirubin, a yellow pigment produced during the normal breakdown of red blood cells. This immaturity of the liver can lead to a buildup of bilirubin in the bloodstream, resulting in jaundice or yellowing of the skin and eyes. As the baby grows and their liver matures, it becomes more efficient in processing and eliminating bilirubin, resolving the hyperbilirubinemia. Therefore, liver immaturity is a key factor in the occurrence of direct hyperbilirubinemia in newborns.

Question 60:

Correct Answer: A) Healthy infant weighing 2500 g, fed 55 cc of expressed human milk via gavage every three hours.

Explanation: Healthy 2500 g infant receiving 55 cc expressed human milk by gavage every 3 hours requires a suitable daily calorie intake. This specific feeding regimen provides important context for determining the appropriate calorie intake for the baby. Expressed human milk is known to be a valuable source of nutrition, containing essential macronutrients, vitamins, and minerals that support the infant's growth and development. By administering 55 cc of expressed human milk every 3 hours, the baby is receiving a consistent and adequate amount of nutrition throughout the day. With this in mind, it can be inferred that the baby's suitable daily calorie intake is being met through this feeding regimen.

Question 61:

Correct Answer: B) Liver

Explanation: The primary site for the biotransformation or metabolism of medications in newborn babies, like little Emma, is the liver. The liver plays a crucial role in the metabolism of drugs as it contains enzymes that help break down medications into smaller, more manageable molecules. These enzymes facilitate the conversion of drugs into metabolites that can be easily eliminated from the body. The liver's ability to metabolize medications is especially important in newborns, as their kidneys are not fully developed and may not be as efficient in excreting drugs. Therefore, the liver takes on the responsibility of metabolizing medications, ensuring their safe elimination from the body.

Question 62:

Correct Answer: A) To stimulate newborn's secretion of insulin

Explanation: Promoting insulin secretion is crucial in preterm newborns with high blood sugar levels. Infusing amino acids serves this purpose by stimulating the release of insulin from the pancreas. Insulin plays a vital role in regulating blood sugar levels by facilitating the uptake of glucose into cells for energy production. By administering amino acids, the body receives essential nutrients necessary for protein synthesis and other metabolic processes. This triggers the release of insulin, which helps normalize blood sugar levels. This approach not only addresses the immediate concern of high blood sugar but also supports the overall growth and development of the preterm newborn.

Question 63:

Correct Answer: B) 3-12 hours after birth

Explanation: Within 3-12 hours after birth, newborn babies diagnosed with neonatal abstinence syndrome (NAS) and experiencing acute alcohol withdrawal are likely to exhibit signs and symptoms. This timeframe is crucial as it marks the onset of withdrawal symptoms in these infants. NAS occurs when a baby is exposed to addictive substances, such as alcohol, during pregnancy. Once the baby is separated from the substance after birth, withdrawal symptoms begin to manifest. These symptoms can include tremors, irritability, excessive crying, feeding difficulties, and even seizures. Therefore, healthcare providers must closely monitor newborns during this critical time to ensure prompt intervention and appropriate management of NAS.

Question 64:

Correct Answer: C) To circumvent the need for intubation and ventilation or to allow for a reduced tidal volume.

Explanation: To avoid intubation and ventilation or permit a lower tidal volume, controlled hypercapnia is utilized as a strategy to prevent bronchopulmonary dysplasia (BPD) or chronic lung disease in neonates. The primary objective behind this approach is to minimize the potential harm caused by invasive mechanical ventilation, which can lead to lung injury and worsen the condition of premature infants. By allowing controlled hypercapnia, healthcare professionals aim to maintain an elevated level of carbon dioxide in the blood within acceptable limits. This technique helps in reducing the need for aggressive ventilation and allows for the use of lower tidal volumes, which are less damaging to the delicate lungs of neonates. Ultimately, the goal is to promote lung development and minimize the risk of BPD or chronic lung disease in these vulnerable infants.

Question 65:

Correct Answer: B) 7 days

Explanation: When the duration of total parenteral nutrition (TPN) is extended to 7 days or more, it is suggested to consider the placement of a central line for its delivery. This is because central lines offer several advantages over peripheral lines for TPN administration. Central lines provide access to larger veins, allowing for the delivery of hypertonic TPN solutions without the risk of peripheral vein irritation or damage. Additionally, central lines can accommodate multiple lumens, facilitating the administration of other essential medications or fluids concurrently with TPN. Moreover, central lines have a lower risk of infection compared to peripheral lines, reducing the likelihood of complications such as catheter-related bloodstream infections. Therefore, based on the extended duration of TPN, the placement of a central line is recommended for optimal delivery and patient safety.

Question 66:

Correct Answer: B) Perform a single suction event before ventilating the neonate.

Explanation: Make only one suction event before ventilating the neonate. This suggested method is based on the principle of minimizing potential harm to the newborn baby during endotracheal suctioning. Performing multiple suction events can lead to excessive and prolonged suctioning, which can cause trauma to the delicate mucosal lining of the trachea and bronchi. Additionally, repeated suctioning can disrupt the baby's breathing pattern and lead to hypoxia or bradycardia. By limiting suctioning to just one event before ventilating, healthcare professionals can effectively clear the airway without subjecting the newborn to unnecessary risks. This approach ensures that the baby's respiratory function is adequately supported while minimizing potential complications associated with excessive suctioning.

Question 67:

Correct Answer: A) Electrolyte imbalance

Explanation: Electrolyte imbalance is NOT considered a possible hazard when utilizing an extracorporeal membrane oxygenation (ECMO) device. Electrolyte imbalance refers to an abnormality in the levels of electrolytes, such as sodium, potassium, calcium, and magnesium, in the body. While ECMO is a complex life support system that involves the use of a pump to oxygenate and circulate blood outside of the body, it does not directly cause electrolyte imbalances. The primary hazards associated with ECMO include bleeding, infection, clotting, mechanical complications, and organ dysfunction. Therefore, it is crucial to monitor and maintain electrolyte balance in patients receiving ECMO, but it is not considered a hazard directly attributable to the device itself.

Question 68:

Correct Answer: B) 2nd and 98th percentiles

Explanation: The cut off values on the World Health Organization (WHO) growth chart that signify abnormal growth are the 2nd and 98th percentiles. These percentiles represent the lower and upper limits, respectively, of what is considered normal growth. The 2nd percentile indicates that only 2% of the population falls below this value, while the 98th percentile suggests that only 2% of the population exceeds this value. Therefore, if a child's growth measurements consistently fall below the 2nd percentile or consistently exceed the 98th percentile, it may indicate abnormal growth patterns. These cut off values serve as important indicators for healthcare professionals to identify potential growth abnormalities and provide appropriate interventions or further evaluations if necessary.

Question 69:

Correct Answer: C) The mass can be diminished through applied pressure.

Explanation: It can be determined that a newborn baby, like baby Anthony, has an inguinal hernia rather than a hydrocele when there is a scrotal mass that can be reduced with pressure. This characteristic is key in distinguishing between the two conditions. In the case of an inguinal hernia, the scrotal mass is caused by a loop of intestine or abdominal tissue that protrudes through a weakness in the abdominal wall. Applying pressure on the mass would result in its reduction back into the abdominal cavity. On the other hand, a hydrocele is a collection of fluid in the scrotum, and applying pressure would not have any effect on its size or consistency. Hence, the ability to reduce the scrotal mass with pressure indicates the presence of an inguinal hernia in baby Anthony.

Question 70:

Correct Answer: C) 10 to 20

Explanation: The usual count of stratum corneum layers found in the epidermis of a full-term newborn is 10 to 20. The stratum corneum is the outermost layer of the epidermis and serves as a protective barrier for the skin. It is composed of multiple layers of flattened, dead skin cells called corneocytes, which are embedded in a lipid-rich matrix. This layer helps to prevent water loss, protect against harmful external agents, and maintain the skin's integrity. In a full-term newborn, the stratum corneum is still developing and may have a lower count of layers compared to adults. However, it gradually increases in thickness and matures over time.

Question 71:

Correct Answer: A) pulse oximeter

Explanation: Pulse oximetry is the most effective method for conducting screening for critical congenital heart disease. This non-invasive and reliable technique measures the oxygen saturation levels in a newborn's blood by using a pulse oximeter. By placing the device on the infant's hand or foot, it can accurately detect any abnormalities in the oxygen levels, indicating the presence of potential heart defects. The simplicity and ease of use make pulse oximetry a preferred choice for screening, as it can be performed quickly and does not cause discomfort to the baby. Additionally, pulse oximetry has demonstrated high sensitivity and specificity in detecting critical congenital heart disease, ensuring early intervention and improved outcomes for affected infants.

Question 72:

Correct Answer: A) Three or more separate fetal movements in 30 minutes

Explanation: Three or more separate fetal movements in 30 minutes is considered a standard rating on the fetal biophysical profile. These criteria is significant as it indicates the presence of fetal well-being and an active, healthy fetus. Fetal movements are an essential indicator of fetal neurologic integrity and overall health. Adequate movements signify that the baby is receiving an adequate oxygen supply and that its central nervous system is developing normally. It is crucial to assess fetal movements as part of the biophysical profile, as changes in movement patterns can be indicative of fetal distress or compromised well-being. Therefore, the presence of three or more separate fetal movements in 30 minutes is considered a reassuring sign and a standard rating on the fetal biophysical profile.

Question 73:

Correct Answer: A) Standard neonatal resuscitation procedures

Explanation: Routine resuscitation steps are the recommended course of action for a newborn if the amniotic fluid is found to be stained with meconium at the time of delivery. Meconium-stained amniotic fluid indicates that the baby may have passed stool before birth, which can increase the risk of respiratory distress and other complications. Therefore, immediate intervention is crucial. The routine resuscitation steps include clearing the airway to remove any meconium present, providing positive pressure ventilation to support breathing, and monitoring the baby's vital signs closely. These steps are aimed at ensuring that the baby receives adequate oxygenation and ventilation, promoting their transition to extrauterine life and reducing the risk of complications associated with meconium aspiration.

Question 74:

Correct Answer: A) Blood or cerebrospinal fluid culture

Explanation: Blood or cerebrospinal fluid culture is the most effective method for diagnosing an early-onset group B streptococcal infection in a newborn. This diagnostic approach involves obtaining a sample of blood or cerebrospinal fluid from the newborn and culturing it in a laboratory setting to identify the presence of the bacteria. The culture allows for the growth and isolation of the group B streptococcus, making it possible to accurately diagnose the infection. By specifically targeting blood or cerebrospinal fluid, this method provides a reliable means of early detection, enabling prompt initiation of appropriate treatment. Other diagnostic methods such as rapid antigen detection tests may offer quicker results but are less sensitive and specific compared to blood or cerebrospinal fluid culture. Therefore, to ensure accurate diagnosis and appropriate management, blood or cerebrospinal fluid culture remains the gold standard for detecting early-onset group B streptococcal infections in newborns.

Question 75:

Correct Answer: B) 3 L/min

Explanation: The initial flow rate for oxygen therapy for a premature neonate weighing 1.4 kg should be 3 L/min. This flow rate is appropriate to provide adequate oxygenation and support for the baby as they transition from the ventilator to nasal high-flow oxygen therapy. Nasal high-flow oxygen therapy is a method of delivering oxygen to the lungs through the nose at a higher flow rate than conventional oxygen therapy. It helps to maintain the baby's airway patency, improve oxygenation, and reduce the work of breathing. By starting with a flow rate of 3 L/min, healthcare professionals ensure that the baby receives the necessary oxygen support while closely monitoring their response. The flow rate may be adjusted based on the baby's oxygen saturation levels and overall clinical condition.

Question 76:

Correct Answer: C) 1.11

Explanation: 1.11 is the conversion factor that should be multiplied by the point-of-care glucose value to estimate the plasma glucose level when performing bedside glucose tests to evaluate low blood sugar levels. This conversion factor takes into account the difference between the glucose levels in whole blood and plasma. Whole blood contains not only glucose but also other components such as red blood cells, white blood cells, and platelets. Plasma, on the other hand, is the liquid part of blood that remains after these components are removed. Since glucose is primarily found in plasma, multiplying the point-of-care glucose value by 1.11 helps adjust for the difference between whole blood and plasma glucose levels, providing a more accurate estimation of the actual plasma glucose level.

Question 77:

Correct Answer: A) PKU is a potentially life-threatening condition, hence its screening is strongly advised.

Explanation: PKU can be a fatal illness and it is highly recommended that this be performed. Phenylketonuria (PKU) is a genetic disorder that affects the body's ability to break down an essential amino acid called phenylalanine. If left untreated, the accumulation of phenylalanine can lead to severe brain damage and intellectual disability in affected individuals. Newborn screening for PKU allows for early detection and intervention, enabling timely treatment to prevent these devastating consequences. By identifying infants with PKU early on, healthcare professionals can provide dietary modifications that restrict phenylalanine intake. This simple intervention helps prevent the buildup of phenylalanine in the body, ensuring normal brain development and allowing affected individuals to lead healthy and fulfilling lives. Therefore, it is crucial for newborns to undergo PKU screening to ensure their well-being and prevent irreversible damage.

Question 78:

Correct Answer: C) 32 to 38 cm

Explanation: The standard head circumference for a newborn baby typically ranges from 32 to 38 cm. This measurement is considered a vital indicator of a baby's growth and development. The variation in head circumference is due to the natural differences in newborn sizes and proportions. It is essential to monitor head circumference regularly during the first few months of life to ensure that the baby's brain and skull are developing properly. Pediatricians use this measurement as part of their routine health assessments to identify any abnormalities or potential issues. Therefore, understanding and tracking the standard range of head circumference is crucial in ensuring the overall well-being of newborns.

Question 79:

Correct Answer: B) All neonates

Explanation: All neonates, or newborns, are recommended by the American Academy of Pediatrics (AAP) to receive Vitamin K shots. This is because newborns have limited amounts of Vitamin K in their bodies, which is necessary for blood clotting. Vitamin K helps prevent a condition called vitamin K deficiency bleeding (VKDB), which can lead to serious bleeding in newborns. By administering Vitamin K shots, the AAP aims to ensure that all neonates have sufficient levels of this essential vitamin to prevent any potential bleeding complications. Therefore, it is crucial for healthcare providers to follow the AAP's recommendation and administer Vitamin K shots to all newborns.

Question 80:

Correct Answer: A) Liam can participate, but he needs to be careful to avoid dehydration or excessive physical exercise.

Explanation: He can participate, but needs to be careful to avoid dehydration or overly strenuous exercise. Sickle cell disease is a condition that affects the shape and function of red blood cells, causing them to become rigid and form a sickle shape. This can block blood flow and oxygen delivery to various organs and tissues in the body. However, engaging in regular sports activities is still possible for individuals with sickle cell disease, including newborns like Liam. It is important for Liam to stay well-hydrated during physical activities to prevent dehydration, which can trigger a sickle cell crisis. Additionally, he should avoid overly strenuous exercise that may put excessive stress on his body and increase the risk of complications. By following these precautions, Liam can still participate in sports activities and lead an active lifestyle.

Question 81:

Correct Answer: C) Toxoplasmosis, rubella, cytomegalovirus, herpes simplex, and other diseases

Explanation: TORCH syndrome refers to a group of infections that can be transmitted from mother to fetus during pregnancy. It encompasses a range of illnesses including Toxoplasmosis, other diseases, rubella, cytomegalovirus, and herpes simplex. Toxoplasmosis is caused by a parasite and can lead to severe complications such as neurological damage. Rubella, commonly known as German measles, can cause birth defects if contracted during pregnancy. Cytomegalovirus (CMV) is a viral infection that can result in developmental issues and hearing loss. Herpes simplex virus can cause serious complications if transmitted to the baby during childbirth. It is crucial for healthcare professionals to be aware of these infections and implement appropriate measures to prevent and manage them during pregnancy.

Question 82:

Correct Answer: A) Record the blood pressure as a normal reading and continue the assessment of the newborn.

Explanation: Record the blood pressure as a normal reading and continue the assessment of the newborn. In the neonatal intensive care setting, it is crucial for nurses to monitor and assess vital signs, including blood pressure, to ensure the well-being of these vulnerable patients. A blood pressure reading of 64/40 may appear low, but it is important to consider the context of the newborn's age and size. Neonates often have lower blood pressure values compared to adults. By recording the blood pressure as a normal reading, the nurse acknowledges that this value falls within the expected range for a newborn. However, it is essential to continue the assessment, as blood pressure alone does not provide a comprehensive picture of the infant's condition. This allows the nurse to identify any other signs or symptoms that may require further intervention or evaluation.

Question 83:

Correct Answer: B) Including estimated data as well as actual data

Explanation: Including estimated data as well as actual data can potentially undermine the validity of conducting clinical research for evidence-based practice. While estimating data can be useful in situations where actual data is unavailable, it is essential to recognize the limitations of estimations. Estimations might introduce bias and inaccuracies, leading to unreliable results. In research, the validity of findings is crucial for informing evidence-based practice decisions. Therefore, relying solely on estimated data without verification through actual data collection and analysis can compromise the accuracy and reliability of the research outcomes. It is imperative to prioritize the use of actual data whenever possible to ensure the validity and credibility of clinical research for evidence-based practice.

Question 84:

Correct Answer: A) 50% of total caloric intake

Explanation: According to medical guidelines, the maximum percentage of total caloric intake that lipids should represent in a parenteral infusate is 50%. Parenteral nutrition is a method of providing essential nutrients intravenously to individuals who are unable to consume food orally. Lipids, such as fats, are a crucial component of parenteral nutrition as they provide a concentrated source of energy. However, it is important to limit the percentage of lipids to 50% of total caloric intake to avoid potential complications. Exceeding this limit can lead to adverse effects like hyperlipidemia and compromised liver function. Therefore, healthcare professionals carefully monitor and regulate the lipid content in parenteral infusates to maintain optimal nutrition and prevent potential risks.

Question 85:

Correct Answer: C) Five

Explanation: Five injections of hyaluronidase are typically administered around the edges of the IV insertion site in the event of an IV medication extravasation. This specific number is determined based on the recommended dosage and administration guidelines of hyaluronidase for the treatment of extravasation. Hyaluronidase is an enzyme that helps to disperse and break down hyaluronic acid, which is responsible for the gel-like consistency of the extracellular matrix. By injecting hyaluronidase around the edges of the IV insertion site, it helps to accelerate the diffusion and absorption of the extravasated medication, reducing the risk of tissue damage and promoting adequate healing. Administering five injections ensures thorough coverage of the affected area and maximizes the effectiveness of the treatment.

Question 86:

Correct Answer: B) SBAR

Explanation: SBAR is a widely recognized mnemonic that stands for Situation, Background, Assessment, and Recommendation. It serves as a guide to ensure effective communication during patient handoff. SBAR provides a structured approach to convey critical information accurately and succinctly. By using SBAR, healthcare professionals can clearly communicate the patient's current situation, including any relevant symptoms or changes in condition (Situation). They then provide a concise background of the patient's medical history, previous interventions, and recent test results (Background). Next, they discuss their assessment of the patient's current status, incorporating vital signs, physical examination findings, and diagnostic data (Assessment). Finally, they offer clear and specific recommendations for ongoing care, including necessary actions or interventions (Recommendation). In summary, SBAR offers a standardized framework that enhances communication, reduces errors, and promotes patient safety during handoffs.

Question 87:

Correct Answer: B) Magnesium

Explanation: Magnesium is a crucial electrolyte that plays a significant role in the development and functioning of the central nervous system. When administered to prematurely born infants, magnesium can effectively lower the risk of neurological impairments. This is because magnesium acts as a neuroprotective agent by reducing the risk of brain injury and minimizing the detrimental effects of hypoxic-ischemic insults. Additionally, magnesium possesses anti-inflammatory properties, which can further contribute to its neuroprotective effects. By maintaining adequate magnesium levels in premature infants, healthcare professionals can enhance neurological outcomes and mitigate the potential long-term complications associated with neurodevelopmental impairments. Overall, the administration of magnesium in prematurely born infants is essential in reducing the risk of neurological impairments and promoting healthy brain development.

Question 88:

Correct Answer: B) The IV is positioned in a region with minimal adipose tissue for optimal vein visibility.

Explanation: The IV needs to be in an area with less fat so the vein can be clearly visualized. This is important because it allows for accurate placement and monitoring of the IV, ensuring that the baby receives the necessary fluids and medications. The scalp is often chosen as the site for IV placement in neonates because the veins in this area are relatively superficial and easily accessible. By placing the IV in the scalp, healthcare professionals can closely monitor the baby's condition and administer treatments as needed. It is understandable that parents may be concerned about this procedure, but they can be reassured that the healthcare team is experienced in neonatal care and will take all necessary precautions to ensure the safety and comfort of their baby.

Question 89:

Correct Answer: B) Biphasic stridor and dyspnea

Explanation: Biphasic stridor and dyspnea are the typical symptoms of tracheal stenosis in a newborn baby. Biphasic stridor refers to a high-pitched, noisy breathing sound that occurs during both the inhalation and exhalation phases. This is caused by the narrowing of the trachea, which obstructs the flow of air and creates turbulence during breathing. Dyspnea, on the other hand, is the medical term for difficulty in breathing. In newborns with tracheal stenosis, dyspnea is often observed as rapid, shallow breathing or increased effort in breathing. These symptoms are crucial indicators of tracheal stenosis and should prompt immediate medical attention to ensure proper diagnosis and timely intervention.

Question 90:

Correct Answer: A) Aorta

Explanation: In the case of the transposition of the great vessels, one important vessel that can be involved is the aorta. The aorta is the largest artery in the body and carries oxygenated blood from the heart to the rest of the body. In transposition of the great vessels, the aorta is positioned incorrectly, arising from the right ventricle instead of the left ventricle. This abnormal positioning leads to a complete reversal of the normal blood flow pattern and can have significant consequences for the circulation. It is important to identify the involvement of the aorta in transposition of the great vessels as it plays a crucial role in carrying oxygenated blood to the body's organs and tissues.

Question 91:

Correct Answer: A) The neonate should be isolated from the mother until her varicella vesicles have crusted over.

Explanation: The neonate must be separated from the mother until the mother's vesicles have dried. This is because varicella, also known as chickenpox, is a highly contagious viral infection that can be transmitted to the newborn if proper precautions are not taken. By separating the newborn from the mother, the risk of transmission is significantly reduced. The drying of the vesicles indicates that the mother is no longer contagious, ensuring the safety of the newborn. It is important to note that newborns have immature immune systems and are more susceptible to infections. Therefore, it is crucial to take all necessary measures to protect them from potential harm.

Question 92:

Correct Answer: A) To the opposite nostril weekly and to a new one monthly

Explanation: To the opposite nostril weekly and to a new one monthly. This recommendation is based on several factors. Firstly, changing the feeding tube to the opposite nostril weekly helps prevent irritation and damage to the nasal passage. By alternating nostrils, the pressure and friction on the same side are reduced, reducing the risk of nasal injury. Secondly, changing the tube to a new nostril monthly helps prevent complications such as infection and blockage. Over time, the build-up of biofilm and debris can occur, leading to infections or tube malfunction. By replacing the tube regularly, the risk of these complications is minimized. Ultimately, adhering to this recommended frequency ensures the long-term polyurethane feeding tubes remain effective and minimizes the potential for adverse events.

Question 93:

Correct Answer: C) Full-term infants

Explanation: Full-term infants are the category where the occurrence of hypoxic ischemic encephalopathy (HIE) is most frequently observed. HIE is a condition characterized by reduced blood flow and oxygen to the brain, leading to potential brain damage. Full-term infants refer to babies who are born between 37 and 42 weeks of gestation. This group is at higher risk for HIE as they have completed the full duration of pregnancy and are more likely to experience complications during labor and delivery. Factors such as prolonged labor, umbilical cord issues, placental abnormalities, or maternal health conditions can contribute to the development of HIE in full-term infants. Therefore, it is crucial to closely monitor and provide immediate medical intervention to this specific category of infants to prevent or minimize the occurrence of HIE.

Question 94:

Correct Answer: A) A germinal matrix hemorrhage

Explanation: A germinal matrix hemorrhage is the term used to describe the least severe type of intraventricular brain hemorrhage in a newborn. This condition occurs when there is bleeding in the area of the brain called the germinal matrix, which is a highly vascular and fragile structure present in premature infants. The germinal matrix is responsible for producing new brain cells and is more susceptible to injury due to its delicate nature. A germinal matrix hemorrhage is considered the least severe type of intraventricular brain hemorrhage because it is confined to the germinal matrix region and does not extend into the ventricles or other areas of the brain. Although it is less severe compared to other types, it still requires careful monitoring and appropriate medical intervention to prevent potential complications.

Question 95:

Correct Answer: B) Cystic fibrosis

Explanation: Cystic fibrosis is a typical example of an autosomal recessive disorder. This genetic condition primarily affects the lungs, pancreas, liver, and intestines. It is caused by mutations in the cystic fibrosis transmembrane conductance regulator (CFTR) gene. Individuals with cystic fibrosis inherit two copies of the mutated CFTR gene, one from each parent. The autosomal recessive inheritance pattern means that both copies of the gene must be mutated for the disease to manifest. Therefore, if an individual carry only one mutated copy of the CFTR gene, they are considered carriers and do not typically exhibit symptoms. Cystic fibrosis is characterized by the production of thick, sticky mucus that can obstruct airways and impair the function of various organs, leading to respiratory and digestive complications.

Question 96:

Correct Answer: C) Congenital adrenal hyperplasia

Explanation: Congenital adrenal hyperplasia (CAH) is the primary reason for unclear genitalia in a newborn girl with typical genetics. CAH is an inherited disorder that affects the adrenal glands, resulting in abnormal levels of certain hormones, such as cortisol and aldosterone. In the case of CAH, there is a deficiency in the enzyme responsible for producing these hormones, leading to an overproduction of androgens (male sex hormones). This excessive androgen production can cause virilization of the female genitalia, leading to ambiguity in the external appearance of the genitalia at birth. Therefore, when evaluating a newborn girl with typical genetics and unclear genitalia, CAH is a crucial consideration.

Question 97:

Correct Answer: C) Regularly change the baby's head position and ensure monitored time on their stomach.

Explanation: Frequently rotating the infant's head and providing supervised tummy time are crucial guidelines that should be given to parents to prevent the occurrence of plagiocephaly or flat head syndrome in their child. Plagiocephaly is often a result of prolonged pressure on a specific area of the baby's skull, which can be caused by consistently placing the infant in the same position. By frequently rotating the baby's head, parents can distribute the pressure evenly and prevent the development of flat spots. Additionally, supervised tummy time allows the infant to strengthen their neck muscles and promotes the natural rounding of the skull. These simple yet effective measures can significantly reduce the risk of plagiocephaly and support the healthy development of the baby's skull.

Question 98:

Correct Answer: B) Cardiac tamponade

Explanation: Cardiac tamponade is a condition characterized by the accumulation of fluid or blood in the pericardial sac, leading to compression of the heart. In the case of a newborn baby with a central venous line, the sudden onset of hemodynamic instability, including pulsus paradoxus, slowed heart rate, subdued heart sounds, and a drop in oxygen saturation despite interventions such as CPAP and increased oxygen flow, could be indicative of cardiac tamponade. This condition hampers the heart's ability to fill and pump effectively, resulting in compromised hemodynamics. It is crucial to recognize and promptly address cardiac tamponade in neonates, as it can rapidly progress to cardiac arrest. Immediate intervention, such as pericardiocentesis or surgical drainage, is essential to alleviate the tamponade and restore normal cardiac function.

Question 99:

Correct Answer: A) Hypocalcemia and hypokalemia

Explanation: Hypocalcemia and hypokalemia are potential conditions that could arise from a lack of magnesium in a newborn's diet. Hypocalcemia refers to low levels of calcium in the blood, which can lead to muscle cramps, seizures, and abnormal heart rhythms. Magnesium plays a crucial role in regulating calcium levels, so a deficiency in magnesium can disrupt this balance and result in hypocalcemia. Similarly, hypokalemia refers to low levels of potassium in the blood. Magnesium is necessary for the proper functioning of potassium channels in cells, and without sufficient magnesium, these channels may not work effectively, leading to reduced potassium levels. Both hypocalcemia and hypokalemia can have serious consequences on a newborn's health and must be addressed promptly.

Question 100:

Correct Answer: C) Late decelerations

Explanation: Late decelerations are a critical indicator of an urgent need for intervention due to insufficient uteroplacental function. These decelerations represent a concerning pattern in fetal heart rate where the heart rate drops significantly and recovers after the contraction. They occur as a result of decreased oxygen supply to the fetus during contractions, suggesting compromised blood flow through the uteroplacental circulation. Late decelerations can be observed during labor and are often associated with conditions such as placental insufficiency or maternal hypertension. Prompt intervention is necessary in such cases to prevent further compromise to the fetus and ensure optimal oxygenation. Monitoring and addressing the underlying cause of late decelerations is crucial to safeguard the well-being of both mother and baby.

Question 101:

Correct Answer: B) 15 to 22

Explanation: The suggested peak inspiratory pressure (PIP) for a neonate once they have been stabilized on ECMO is 15 to 22. This range is recommended to maintain adequate oxygenation and ventilation while minimizing the risk of lung injury in neonates undergoing ECMO therapy. The PIP is carefully titrated based on the individual patient's needs, taking into consideration factors such as lung compliance, oxygenation levels, and the severity of lung disease. It is important to closely monitor the neonate's response to the set PIP and make adjustments as needed to optimize their respiratory support. By maintaining PIP within the suggested range, clinicians can provide optimal respiratory support for neonates on ECMO while minimizing the risk of complications.

Question 102:

Correct Answer: A) Persistent crying

Explanation: Persistent crying is not considered an early sign of hunger in a newborn. While crying is a common way for infants to communicate their needs, it is not necessarily an indicator of hunger in the early stages. Newborns typically exhibit other signs of hunger before resorting to crying, such as smacking their lips, rooting, or making sucking motions. These cues are often subtle and can be easily missed if not closely observed. Therefore, it is important for caregivers to pay attention to these early hunger cues to ensure prompt feeding and prevent excessive crying or distress in the newborn.

Question 103:

Correct Answer: B) Bradycardia and decreased fetal heart rate variability

Explanation: Bradycardia and decreased fetal heart rate variability are the usual impacts on the baby when a soon-to-be mother, such as Mrs. Michaelson, is given magnesium sulfate as a tocolytic to extend her pregnancy. Magnesium sulfate is commonly used to relax the uterine muscles and delay preterm labor. However, it can also cross the placenta and affect the baby's cardiovascular system. Bradycardia refers to a slower than normal heart rate in the fetus, while decreased fetal heart rate variability indicates a reduced fluctuation in the baby's heart rate. These effects occur due to the suppressive action of magnesium sulfate on the baby's central nervous system. Monitoring the fetal heart rate and promptly adjusting the dosage of magnesium sulfate is essential to ensure the well-being of both the mother and the baby during this intervention.

Question 104:

Correct Answer: C) 1 cc pediatric acetaminophen liquid, orally every 6 hours

Explanation: 1 cc of pediatric acetaminophen liquid, orally every 6 hours would be the most suitable dosage for managing Jacob's pain following his circumcision procedure. Acetaminophen is a commonly used medication for pain relief in infants. The recommended dosage for infants is based on their weight, and Jacob, weighing 6 lbs, falls within the appropriate range for this dosage. The oral route of administration is preferred for infants as it is easy to administer and provides effective pain relief. By giving Jacob 1 cc of pediatric acetaminophen liquid every 6 hours, we can ensure that he receives the appropriate amount of medication to manage his pain without exceeding the recommended dosage. It is important to follow the prescribed dosage and consult with a healthcare professional for any concerns or questions regarding the use of acetaminophen in infants.

Question 105:

Correct Answer: C) The neonate has a normal head circumference but below-normal weight.

Explanation: When a newborn is categorized as asymmetrically small for gestational age (SGA), it implies that the neonate has a normal head circumference but below-normal weight. This condition indicates that the baby's growth has been restricted during pregnancy, resulting in a lower birth weight compared to what is expected for its gestational age. The term "asymmetrically" refers to the fact that the baby's head circumference is within the normal range, suggesting that the restriction in growth primarily affects the body, rather than the head. This distinction is important as it helps in identifying the underlying causes and potential complications associated with SGA.

Question 106:

Correct Answer: C) Short-gut syndrome

Explanation: Short-gut syndrome is a condition that may require the administration of total parenteral nutrition (TPN). This condition occurs when a significant portion of the small intestine has been surgically removed or is non-functional due to disease or injury. As a result, the body is unable to absorb nutrients properly, leading to malnutrition and weight loss. TPN, which is the delivery of nutrients intravenously, bypasses the digestive system and provides the necessary nutrients directly into the bloodstream. It is an essential treatment option for individuals with short-gut syndrome, as it ensures that their nutritional needs are met while allowing the intestines to heal. By supporting the body's nutritional requirements, TPN plays a crucial role in improving the overall health and well-being of patients with short-gut syndrome.

Question 107:

Correct Answer: C) Post the second year of existence

Explanation: After the second year of life, a child diagnosed with late congenital syphilis would typically begin to exhibit symptoms. Late congenital syphilis refers to the manifestation of the disease in children who were infected with syphilis during pregnancy but did not show symptoms at birth. It is important to note that the initial signs of late congenital syphilis can be subtle and easily overlooked, which makes early detection and treatment crucial. Common symptoms that may indicate late congenital syphilis include bone deformities, such as saddle nose or saber shins, as well as dental abnormalities and hearing loss. Prompt diagnosis and intervention are essential to prevent further complications and ensure the child's well-being.

Question 108:

Correct Answer: B) Administer the aspirate back and proceed with the feeding.

Explanation: Refeeding the aspirate and carrying out the feeding would be the most suitable course of action in this scenario. When the aspirate contains roughly 40% of the previous feeding that hasn't been fully digested, it indicates a potential delay in gastric emptying or impaired digestion. By refeeding the aspirate, we are essentially reintroducing the undigested portion back into the stomach for further processing. This allows for a more complete digestion and absorption of nutrients. Once the aspirate has been re-fed, it is important to proceed with the planned feeding to ensure that the patient receives the necessary nutrition. This approach minimizes the risk of malnutrition and ensures optimal nutrient utilization.

Question 109:

Correct Answer: A) 32 to 36 weeks of gestation

Explanation: During the developmental process, it is typical for a baby, like little Emma, to shed her lanugo between 32 to 36 weeks of gestation. Lanugo refers to the fine, downy hair that covers a baby's body in the womb. This hair serves as a protective layer and helps to regulate their body temperature. However, as the baby approaches the final stages of gestation, the lanugo starts to diminish. By the 32nd to 36th week, most of the lanugo is shed, making way for the growth of more mature hair, such as the hair on the scalp. This shedding of lanugo is a natural part of the baby's development and signifies their readiness for life outside the womb.

Question 110:

Correct Answer: A) Hirschsprung's disease

Explanation: Hirschsprung's disease is a potential issue that could explain the symptoms of a newborn baby who hasn't had a bowel movement in the first two days of life and has been vomiting after every oral feeding. This condition is characterized by the absence of nerve cells in certain segments of the bowel, leading to a lack of proper bowel movements. The affected portion of the intestine becomes blocked, causing a buildup of stool and subsequent distension. This can result in the inability to pass stool, leading to constipation and abdominal distention. Additionally, the blockage can cause the stomach to empty poorly, resulting in vomiting after feeding. Identifying Hirschsprung's disease is crucial as it requires surgical intervention to remove the affected portion of the bowel and restore normal digestive function.

Question 111:

Correct Answer: B) Peritoneal fluid culture

Explanation: Peritoneal fluid culture is the recommended diagnostic procedure to guide the therapeutic approach for spontaneous intestinal perforation (FIP). This procedure involves the collection and analysis of fluid from the peritoneal cavity, which surrounds the abdominal organs. By analyzing the peritoneal fluid, clinicians can identify the presence of bacteria or other pathogens that may be causing the intestinal perforation. This information is crucial for determining the appropriate course of treatment, such as selecting the most effective antibiotics or considering surgical intervention. Peritoneal fluid culture provides valuable insights into the specific infectious agents involved in FIP, allowing healthcare professionals to tailor their therapeutic approach accordingly.

Question 112:

Correct Answer: B)Fats and calcium

Explanation: Fats and calcium are two essential nutrients that may be excessively lost due to continuous gavage feedings. Gavage feedings, which involve the administration of nutrients directly into the stomach through a tube, can result in increased fat malabsorption. This is because fats require certain enzymes and bile acids for proper digestion and absorption, which may be compromised in individuals receiving gavage feedings. Additionally, continuous gavage feedings can also lead to calcium loss. Calcium is primarily absorbed in the small intestine, and the rapid delivery of nutrients through gavage feedings may disrupt this process. Furthermore, certain medications used in gavage feedings, such as acid-reducing drugs, can further interfere with calcium absorption. Therefore, it is crucial to closely monitor and supplement fats and calcium in individuals receiving continuous gavage feedings to prevent deficiencies and ensure optimal nutritional status.

Question 113:

Correct Answer: B) Hydration, electrolyte supplementation, and initiation of parenteral nutrition

Explanation: Hydration, electrolyte supplementation, and initiation of parenteral nutrition are the initial steps in the nutritional management of short bowel syndrome following a resection due to necrotizing enterocolitis (NEC). Hydration is crucial to restore and maintain optimal fluid balance, as patients with short bowel syndrome are at risk of dehydration due to increased fluid losses. Electrolyte supplementation is necessary to correct any electrolyte imbalances that may have occurred as a result of the resection. Initiation of parenteral nutrition is essential to provide the necessary nutrients and calories to support the patient's growth and development. As the remaining bowel may not be able to adequately absorb nutrients, parenteral nutrition delivers nutrients directly into the bloodstream, bypassing the gastrointestinal tract. These initial steps aim to stabilize the patient's fluid and electrolyte status while providing essential nutrition, forming the foundation for further nutritional management in individuals with short bowel syndrome following NEC resection.

Question 114:

Correct Answer: C) Renal function

Explanation: Renal function is the crucial aspect that needs to be closely monitored when a newborn baby is being treated for meningitis with gentamicin. Gentamicin is an antibiotic commonly used to treat infections, including meningitis, in newborns. However, it is known to have potential nephrotoxicity, meaning it can cause damage to the kidneys. Therefore, it is essential to closely monitor the baby's renal function throughout the treatment course. This involves assessing kidney function through laboratory tests, such as measuring serum creatinine levels and monitoring urine output. By closely monitoring renal function, healthcare professionals can detect early signs of kidney damage and take appropriate measures to prevent further complications.

Question 115:

Correct Answer: A) A premature infant being formula fed

Explanation: Necrotizing enterocolitis (NEC) is a serious medical condition that primarily affects premature infants. Among them, those who are being formula fed are at the highest risk of contracting NEC. The immature gastrointestinal tract of premature infants is ill-equipped to handle the challenges of formula feeding. Formula contains complex proteins that can be difficult to digest and may lead to an overgrowth of harmful bacteria in the intestines. This can subsequently result in inflammation and damage to the intestinal lining, leading to NEC. Breast milk, on the other hand, provides essential nutrients and protective factors that aid in the development of a healthy gut. Therefore, it is crucial to prioritize breast milk feeding for premature infants to minimize the risk of NEC.

Question 116:

Correct Answer: B) Abruptio placentae

Explanation: Abruptio placentae refer to the premature separation of the placenta from the uterine wall, resulting in a deprivation of oxygen and nutrients for the fetus. This condition can occur in various scenarios, such as trauma to the abdomen, high blood pressure, smoking, drug use, or a previous history of placental abruption. The separation of the placenta can lead to significant bleeding, which can be concealed or visible. This detachment disrupts the normal blood flow between the mother and fetus, compromising the delivery of vital nutrients and oxygen to the baby. Prompt medical intervention is crucial to manage the potential risks to both the mother and the fetus in such cases.

Question 117:

Correct Answer: B) Vastus lateralis/anterolateral thigh

Explanation: Vastus lateralis, also known as the anterolateral thigh, is the ideal site for administering an intramuscular injection in both preterm and full-term newborns. This site is chosen for several reasons. Firstly, the vastus lateralis muscle is well-developed and easily accessible in newborns, making it a suitable location for injection. Secondly, using this site minimizes the risk of injury to vital structures such as nerves and blood vessels. Additionally, the vastus lateralis muscle has a relatively large muscle mass, allowing for better absorption and distribution of the medication. Lastly, this site provides a sufficient distance from major joints, reducing the risk of joint injury. Therefore, healthcare providers should consider the vastus lateralis/anterolateral thigh as the preferred site for intramuscular injections in newborns.

Question 118:

Correct Answer: B) Volvulus

Explanation: Volvulus is the gut disorder that can potentially develop due to malrotation. Volvulus occurs when the bowel twists around itself, leading to a blockage and impaired blood supply. Malrotation refers to the abnormal positioning of the intestines during fetal development. This condition can result in the intestines becoming twisted or kinked, causing volvulus. Volvulus can be a life-threatening condition as it can lead to bowel obstruction, ischemia, and necrosis. Symptoms may include severe abdominal pain, distention, vomiting, and bloody stools. Prompt medical intervention is crucial to relieve the obstruction and restore blood flow to the affected area, usually through surgical correction.

Question 119:

Correct Answer: C) 48 hours

Explanation: The initiation of early oral feedings for newborns who are receiving tube feedings is recommended to commence after 48 hours. This time frame allows for the newborn to undergo a period of adaptation and stabilization, ensuring their readiness for oral intake. The 48-hour mark takes into consideration the physiological changes that occur during the first few days of life, such as the maturation of the gastrointestinal system and the establishment of appropriate sucking and swallowing reflexes. Starting oral feedings at this stage promotes the development of a coordinated feeding pattern, reducing the risk of complications and facilitating the transition from tube to oral feeding. Therefore, a 48-hour period is considered optimal for initiating early oral feedings in newborns who are on tube feedings.

Question 120:

Correct Answer: C) Kidney function and platelet count

Explanation: Kidney function and platelet count are two crucial laboratory examinations that should be closely observed in a newborn baby who has been treated with indomethacin for a patent ductus arteriosus (PDA). Indomethacin, a nonsteroidal anti-inflammatory drug, is commonly used to close a PDA. However, it can have potential adverse effects on the kidneys and platelets. Monitoring kidney function is essential as indomethacin can cause renal impairment, leading to decreased urine output or elevated levels of creatinine. Similarly, platelet count should be closely monitored as indomethacin can induce platelet dysfunction or thrombocytopenia. Regular monitoring of these parameters allows for early detection of any abnormalities and prompt intervention if needed, ensuring the safety and well-being of the newborn baby.

Question 121:

Correct Answer: C) Cystic fibrosis

Explanation: Cystic fibrosis is the most likely condition that Jack, a newborn baby suffering from meconium ileus, is dealing with. Cystic fibrosis is a genetic disorder that affects the lungs, digestive system, and other organs. Meconium ileus, a condition characterized by the blockage of the small intestine with thick, sticky meconium, is a common manifestation of cystic fibrosis in newborns. The thickened meconium is a result of the malfunctioning of the exocrine glands, which secrete abnormally thick mucus. This mucus obstructs the intestines, leading to meconium ileus. It is essential to diagnose cystic fibrosis early to initiate appropriate management and prevent further complications.

Question 122:

Correct Answer: C) Fetal macrosomia

Explanation: Fetal macrosomia is a condition that affects approximately half of the babies born to mothers with diabetes. It is characterized by excessive fetal growth and larger-than-average birth weight. This condition occurs because high levels of glucose in the mother's blood can cross the placenta and stimulate the baby's pancreas to produce more insulin. This excess insulin promotes the storage of glucose as fat, leading to increased fetal growth. Fetal macrosomia poses several risks during childbirth, such as shoulder dystocia and birth injuries. Additionally, babies with this condition are more likely to develop long-term health complications, including obesity and type 2 diabetes later in life. Therefore, it is crucial for mothers with diabetes to closely manage their blood sugar levels to reduce the risk of fetal macrosomia and its associated complications.

Question 123:

Correct Answer: B) Administer a pacifier for the infant to suck on during tube feedings.

Explanation: To assist Liam, the premature baby, in transitioning from tube feeding to oral feeding, a helpful approach would be to introduce a pacifier during his tube feedings. Giving him a pacifier to suck on during the tube feedings can aid in developing his sucking reflex and oral motor skills, which are crucial for successful oral feeding. The pacifier provides the baby with an opportunity to practice the coordination and strength required for sucking, swallowing, and breathing. This practice helps to stimulate the baby's natural feeding instincts, making the transition to oral feeding smoother and more efficient. Additionally, sucking on a pacifier can provide comfort and soothing for Liam, creating a positive association with feeding and reducing potential feeding aversions.

Question 124:

Correct Answer: C) 6 weeks

Explanation: At approximately 6 weeks of age, newborn babies typically gain the ability to lift their head while lying on their stomach. This milestone is an important indication of the baby's developing neck strength and control. At this stage, the muscles in their neck and upper body begin to strengthen, allowing them to gradually raise their head off the surface. This ability is crucial for the baby's overall motor development and prepares them for future milestones such as rolling over, sitting up, and eventually crawling. It is important to note that each baby develops at their own pace, so some may achieve this milestone a little earlier or later than others.

Question 125:

Correct Answer: B) Stage 2

Explanation: Stage 2 of hypoxic-ischemic encephalopathy (HIE) is when a patient, like Thomas, may potentially experience seizures. During this stage, which typically occurs within 6 to 48 hours after the initial insult, the brain undergoes significant metabolic changes due to the lack of oxygen and blood flow. These changes can lead to the release of excitatory neurotransmitters and the development of abnormal electrical activity in the brain, resulting in seizures. Seizures in Stage 2 of HIE are often characterized by repetitive movements, changes in muscle tone, and altered consciousness. Prompt identification and management of seizures in this stage are crucial to prevent further brain injury and improve long-term outcomes for patients like Thomas.

Question 126:

Correct Answer: B) PPHN (persistent pulmonary hypertension of the newborn)

Explanation: PPHN (persistent pulmonary hypertension of the newborn) is a severe consequence related to meconium aspiration in a newborn baby. Meconium aspiration occurs when a baby inhales meconium, the baby's first stool, into their lungs during or before delivery. This can lead to the obstruction of the airways and cause respiratory distress. PPHN is a condition where the blood vessels in the lungs don't relax properly, resulting in increased pressure in the pulmonary arteries. This can lead to decreased oxygen levels in the blood, which can be life-threatening for the baby. PPHN requires immediate medical attention and treatment, including oxygen therapy and mechanical ventilation, to help the baby breathe and stabilize their condition.

Question 127:

Correct Answer: A) Staphylococcus aureus

Explanation: Staphylococcus aureus is the primary cause of nosocomial infections in full-term newborns. This bacterium is a common resident of the nasal cavity and skin of healthy individuals, making it easily transmissible in a hospital environment. The immature immune system of newborns makes them particularly susceptible to infections. Staphylococcus aureus can enter their bodies through invasive procedures, contaminated medical devices, or close contact with healthcare personnel. Once inside, it can cause a range of infections, including skin and soft tissue infections, bloodstream infections, and pneumonia. The ability of Staphylococcus aureus to develop resistance to antibiotics further complicates treatment options, making it crucial to implement strict infection control measures in neonatal units to minimize the risk of transmission.

Question 128:

Correct Answer: A) II

Explanation: II. The classification grade assigned to an intraventricular hemorrhage that has extended into 10% to 40% of the lateral ventricles, without causing significant dilation, is Grade II. Grade II intraventricular hemorrhages are characterized by blood filling less than 50% of the ventricular system without any ventricular enlargement. This classification indicates a moderate level of bleeding within the ventricles. Although there is involvement of a significant portion of the lateral ventricles, the absence of significant dilation suggests that the hemorrhage has not caused severe pressure effects or obstructed the normal cerebrospinal fluid flow. Early identification and monitoring of Grade II intraventricular hemorrhages are crucial to prevent potential complications and ensure appropriate management.

Question 129:

Correct Answer: A) Administration of Caffeine and usage of CPAP

Explanation: Caffeine and CPAP are the typical treatment approaches for a newborn suffering from mixed-type Apnea of Prematurity (AOP). Caffeine, a respiratory stimulant, is administered orally or intravenously to stimulate the central nervous system, improve lung function, and reduce the incidence of apnea episodes in premature infants. It helps in the maturation of the respiratory centers in the brain, thus reducing the episodes of apnea. CPAP (Continuous Positive Airway Pressure) is another crucial treatment method for AOP. It involves delivering a constant flow of air or oxygen through the infant's nostrils, which helps keep the airway open and maintain adequate lung expansion. CPAP therapy prevents the collapse of the airways during expiration, ensuring a continuous flow of oxygen to the lungs and reducing the severity and frequency of apnea events. Combining caffeine and CPAP therapy has proven to be effective in managing mixed-type AOP in newborns. The caffeine helps stimulate the respiratory centers in the brain, while CPAP ensures a stable airway and optimal lung function. This combined approach improves the respiratory status of premature infants, reduces the need for invasive interventions like intubation and mechanical ventilation, and promotes better overall outcomes.

Question 130:

Correct Answer: C) The protein content is higher in colostrum than in mature milk.

Explanation: The protein content is higher in colostrum than in mature milk. This difference can be attributed to the unique composition of colostrum, which is specifically designed to provide essential nutrients and immune factors to newborns. Colostrum is rich in proteins such as immunoglobulins, lactoferrin, and cytokines, which play crucial roles in protecting the infant against infections and supporting their developing immune system. These proteins are present in high concentrations during the initial days after birth, gradually decreasing as the milk transitions to mature milk. On the other hand, mature human milk contains a lower protein content but still provides a balanced and adequate amount of proteins for the continued growth and development of the infant.

Question 131:

Correct Answer: B) Extrahepatic biliary atresia

Explanation: Extrahepatic biliary atresia (EBA) is a potential reason for a newborn baby to experience direct hyperbilirubinemia. EBA is a rare congenital disorder characterized by the absence or obstruction of the bile ducts outside the liver. This obstruction prevents the normal flow of bile, leading to the accumulation of bilirubin in the blood. As a result, the baby's skin and eyes may appear yellowish, a condition known as jaundice. EBA typically presents within the first few weeks of life and requires prompt medical intervention, such as a surgical procedure called the Kasai procedure, to establish biliary drainage. Early detection and management of EBA are crucial to prevent long-term complications and ensure the baby's well-being.

Question 132:

Correct Answer: B) Liver immaturity

Explanation: Liver immaturity is typically the primary reason for direct hyperbilirubinemia in a newborn baby. During the first few days of life, the liver of a newborn is still developing and may not be able to efficiently process bilirubin, a yellow pigment produced from the breakdown of red blood cells. This leads to an accumulation of bilirubin in the blood, resulting in jaundice. The immature liver lacks the necessary enzymes to conjugate bilirubin, making it difficult for the body to eliminate it through the usual pathways. Consequently, the excess bilirubin can build up in the skin and other tissues, leading to the characteristic yellow discoloration. While there can be other causes for direct hyperbilirubinemia, such as liver diseases or infections, liver immaturity is the most common reason in newborns.

Question 133:

Correct Answer: A) <<32 weeks

Explanation: Intraventricular hemorrhage (IVH) primarily affects neonates in the gestational age group of <<32 weeks. IVH refers to bleeding within the ventricles of the brain, which can occur in premature infants due to the fragility of their blood vessels. The risk of IVH is highest in extremely preterm infants, typically those born before 32 weeks of gestation. This is because the blood vessels in the brain of premature babies are not fully developed and are more prone to rupture. IVH can have serious consequences, leading to long-term neurodevelopmental issues. Therefore, it is crucial to provide appropriate care and monitoring for neonates in this gestational age group to mitigate the risk of IVH and its potential complications.

Question 134:

Correct Answer: B) Flushing

Explanation: Flushing is the body's automatic reaction to stress. It is a physiological response triggered by the release of stress hormones, particularly adrenaline. When we experience stress, our body's fight-or-flight response is activated, preparing us to either face the stressor or run away from it. As a part of this response, our blood vessels dilate, increasing blood flow to the skin's surface. This increased blood flow causes flushing, characterized by a reddening of the skin. Flushing is an essential adaptive mechanism that ensures an adequate supply of nutrients and oxygen to the muscles and organs during times of stress. It is just one of the many ways our body responds to stress, alongside increased heart rate, heightened senses, and the release of cortisol.

Question 135 :

Correct Answer: C) Respiratory distress syndrome

Explanation: RDS (respiratory distress syndrome) is typically the primary reason for the occurrence of pneumothorax in newborn babies. RDS is a common condition in premature infants, characterized by underdeveloped lungs and insufficient surfactant production. Surfactant is a substance that helps the lungs expand and prevents their collapse. In the absence of adequate surfactant, the air sacs in the lungs can become stiff and collapsed, leading to difficulty in breathing. As a result, babies with RDS often require mechanical ventilation or other respiratory support. Unfortunately, the use of positive pressure ventilation can sometimes cause air to leak into the space between the lungs and the chest wall, resulting in pneumothorax. Therefore, in newborn babies, RDS is the primary underlying cause of pneumothorax. Respiratory distress syndrome

Question 136:

Correct Answer: C) Vitamin A

Explanation: Vitamin A is the recommended vitamin to administer to newborns that are susceptible to developing bronchopulmonary dysplasia (BPD). This essential nutrient plays a crucial role in lung development and function. Vitamin A promotes the growth and differentiation of respiratory epithelial cells, enhances surfactant production, and helps maintain the integrity of lung tissue. Additionally, it has antioxidant properties that protect against lung injury and inflammation. Studies have shown that vitamin A supplementation in preterm infants reduces the incidence and severity of BPD. Therefore, providing newborns at risk of developing BPD with vitamin A can support their lung development and minimize the risk of respiratory complications.

Question 137:

Correct Answer: A) Ensure the presence of an interpreter proficient in medical terminology.

Explanation: Arrange to have an interpreter familiar with medical terminology present. This is the most effective method to communicate with a patient like Maria and her non-English speaking family. It is crucial to have an interpreter who not only understands the language but also has knowledge of medical terminology to ensure accurate and clear communication. An interpreter will bridge the language barrier, enabling healthcare professionals to explain medical conditions, discuss treatment options, and address any concerns effectively. This approach ensures that Maria and her family fully comprehend the information, actively participate in decision-making, and have their questions answered. It promotes patient-centered care, enhances trust, and reduces the risk of misunderstandings or medical errors. Thus, arranging for a qualified interpreter is vital for effective communication in this scenario.

Question 138:

Correct Answer: C) The likelihood of enduring fertility complications due to this condition is extremely minimal.

Explanation: There is a very low chance of this causing any fertility issues long-term. Neonatal testicular torsion, resulting in one testicle being beyond repair, while the other remains unaffected, is a rare condition that typically occurs in newborn boys. Although the loss of one testicle may have some impact on hormone production, the remaining testicle is usually able to compensate adequately. It is important to note that fertility is a complex process that involves various factors beyond the presence of both testicles. Factors such as sperm count, motility, and overall reproductive health also play a significant role. Therefore, it is highly unlikely that this condition will have a significant impact on the baby boy's ability to have children in the future. It is advisable for the parents to consult with a urologist or reproductive specialist who can provide more specific information and guidance based on the individual case.

Question 139:

Correct Answer: C) Endotracheal

Explanation: Endotracheal administration is not advised for giving naloxone (Narcan) to babies. The rationale behind this recommendation is that endotracheal administration of naloxone may not be as effective as other methods in infants. Naloxone is an opioid antagonist used to reverse the effects of opioid overdose. It works by blocking the opioid receptors in the brain. However, when administered endotracheally, the absorption and distribution of naloxone may be inconsistent and unpredictable in infants, leading to suboptimal reversal of opioid effects. Therefore, alternative routes of administration, such as intravenous or intranasal, are preferred in infants to ensure prompt and effective reversal of opioid overdose.

Question 140:

Correct Answer: B) Atrial-septal defect

Explanation: Atrial-septal defect (ASD) is the most frequent heart irregularity observed in individuals with Trisomy 18. This condition is characterized by a hole in the wall (septum) that separates the two upper chambers of the heart, known as the atria. ASD occurs due to incomplete closure of the atrial septum during fetal development. The presence of Trisomy 18 further increases the likelihood of developing this defect. ASD can lead to abnormal blood flow between the atria, causing strain on the heart and reducing its overall efficiency. This heart irregularity is significant as it can contribute to the cardiovascular complications commonly seen in individuals with Trisomy 18, impacting their overall health and well-being.

Question 141:

Correct Answer: B) NAS may result from the neonate's iatrogenic exposure to opiates intended for sedation or analgesia.

Explanation: NAS can be caused by iatrogenic exposure of opiates to the neonate for the purpose of sedation and/or analgesia. This means that when a pregnant woman uses opiates during pregnancy, the baby can become dependent on these substances. After birth, the baby experiences withdrawal symptoms as the drugs leave their system, leading to the development of NAS. The severity of NAS can vary depending on various factors such as the type and amount of drug exposure, the duration of drug use during pregnancy, and individual factors of the baby. It is crucial for healthcare professionals to identify and manage NAS promptly to ensure the well-being of the affected newborns.

Question 142:

Correct Answer: C) Gastroenteritis

Explanation: Gastroenteritis is a highly contagious condition that affects the gastrointestinal tract, causing symptoms such as diarrhea, vomiting, and abdominal pain. Due to its contagious nature, it is advised to either provide a private room or group together patients suffering from the same infection in a medical setting. This precautionary measure aims to prevent the spread of the infection to other patients and healthcare workers. By isolating patients with gastroenteritis, the risk of transmission through direct contact or contaminated surfaces is significantly reduced. Additionally, grouping infected patients together allows for more efficient monitoring and implementation of infection control measures, such as enhanced hand hygiene and environmental cleaning. Ultimately, this approach helps to minimize the potential spread of gastroenteritis within the medical setting and safeguard the well-being of both patients and healthcare providers.

Question 143:

Correct Answer: B) Gavage feeding

Explanation: Gavage feeding, also known as tube feeding, is the recommended approach to nourish a prematurely born baby like little Emma who has a feeble sucking reflex. Gavage feeding involves the administration of breast milk or formula through a small tube inserted through the nose or mouth directly into the stomach. This method ensures that the baby receives adequate nutrition and hydration while bypassing the need for a strong sucking reflex. Gavage feeding allows for precise control of the amount and rate of feeding, reducing the risk of aspiration and promoting optimal growth and development. It is a safe and effective approach that provides the necessary nutrients for premature infants who have difficulty feeding orally.

Question 144:

Correct Answer: B) Short bowel syndrome

Explanation: Short bowel syndrome is a medical condition that may require the ongoing use of total parenteral nutrition (TPN). This condition occurs when a significant portion of the small intestine is surgically removed or is dysfunctional, leading to a reduced ability to absorb nutrients and fluids from the diet. As a result, patients with short bowel syndrome often struggle to maintain adequate nutrition and hydration through oral intake alone. TPN, a method of providing nutrients intravenously, becomes necessary to ensure the patient's nutritional needs are met. By bypassing the gastrointestinal tract, TPN allows for direct delivery of essential nutrients, including carbohydrates, proteins, fats, vitamins, and minerals, into the bloodstream. Consequently, short bowel syndrome patients can receive the necessary nutrition to support their health and well-being.

Question 145:

Correct Answer: A) Interprofessional practice

Explanation: Interprofessional practice, also known as collaborative care, is the term used to describe the model of care in the Neonatal Intensive Care Unit (NICU) where neonates are looked after by a collaborative team comprising of nurses, doctors, respiratory therapists, and occupational therapists. This approach emphasizes the importance of a multidisciplinary team working together to provide comprehensive and holistic care to neonates. Interprofessional practice recognizes that each healthcare professional brings unique skills and expertise to the table, and by working collaboratively, they can optimize patient outcomes and improve the overall quality of care. In the NICU, this model of care ensures that neonates receive the specialized attention they require from a diverse team of healthcare professionals, promoting the best possible outcomes for these vulnerable patients.

Question 146:

Correct Answer: C) Inappropriate positioning and latching on

Explanation: Inappropriate positioning and latching on are typically the primary reasons for experiencing discomfort in the nipples for a mother who is breastfeeding. When a baby doesn't latch on properly or the mother's position is incorrect, it can lead to nipple pain and discomfort. Inadequate latch can result in the baby not grasping the entire nipple and areola, causing friction and soreness. This can further lead to cracked or bleeding nipples, which can be extremely painful for the mother. Ensuring a correct latch and positioning can alleviate discomfort and promote effective breastfeeding. Seeking guidance from a lactation consultant or healthcare professional can greatly help in resolving these issues and ensuring a positive breastfeeding experience for both the mother and baby.

Question 147:

Correct Answer: B) An opening between the pulmonary and aortic arteries

Explanation: Patent ductus arteriosus refers to an opening between the pulmonary and aortic arteries. This condition occurs when the ductus arteriosus, which is a blood vessel that connects these two arteries during fetal development, fails to close after birth. The ductus arteriosus is essential for fetal circulation, allowing blood to bypass the non-functioning lungs. However, it should close shortly after birth to redirect blood flow to the lungs for oxygenation. When this opening remains, it leads to a persistent shunting of blood from the aorta to the pulmonary artery, causing excessive blood flow to the lungs. If left untreated, patent ductus arteriosus can lead to various complications, such as heart failure and pulmonary hypertension.

Question 148:

Correct Answer: A) Shared decision making

Explanation: Shared decision making is the most accurate description of a situation where the parents of a newborn baby in the Neonatal Intensive Care Unit (NICU) are present at every infant care meeting and actively contribute to all care-related decisions. This approach to healthcare decision making recognizes the importance of including parents as equal partners in the decision-making process. By involving parents in discussions, healthcare professionals can benefit from their unique knowledge and insights about their baby's individual needs and preferences. This collaborative process fosters a sense of empowerment and trust between the healthcare team and the parents, ultimately leading to more informed and personalized care decisions for the newborn. Shared decision making in the NICU setting ensures that the best interests of the baby are prioritized while respecting the values and preferences of the parents.

Question 149:

Correct Answer: B) 0.2 g/kg/hr

Explanation: The maximum speed at which fat emulsions for parenteral nutrition should be given is 0.2 g/kg/hr. This rate is determined based on several factors such as patient tolerance and safety considerations. Fat emulsions are an essential component of parenteral nutrition, providing a concentrated source of calories and essential fatty acids. However, administering fat emulsions at a rapid rate can overwhelm the body's ability to handle the excess fat load, potentially leading to complications such as hypertriglyceridemia and liver dysfunction. Therefore, it is crucial to adhere to the recommended maximum speed of 0.2 g/kg/hr to ensure patient safety and optimize the effectiveness of parenteral nutrition therapy.

Question 150:

Correct Answer: C) Associated anomalies

Explanation: Associated anomalies are a crucial aspect to consider when evaluating a newborn, such as baby Mia, who has been diagnosed with an omphalocele. This condition, characterized by the presence of abdominal organs protruding through the umbilical cord, is often associated with other congenital abnormalities. Therefore, additional evaluations should be conducted to identify any potential complications or associated conditions. These evaluations may include a comprehensive physical examination, genetic testing, and imaging studies such as ultrasounds or X-rays. By carefully assessing for associated anomalies, healthcare professionals can ensure a comprehensive understanding of the newborn's overall health status and provide appropriate management and interventions as needed.

Question 151:

Correct Answer: A) Reactive hypoglycemia

Explanation: Reactive hypoglycemia is a possible outcome if the glucose intake of a newborn, who is on parenteral nutrition, is decreased too rapidly. Reactive hypoglycemia refers to a condition in which blood sugar levels drop to abnormally low levels after a meal or a sudden decrease in glucose intake. In the case of a newborn relying on parenteral nutrition, any sudden reduction in glucose supply could disrupt the delicate balance of blood sugar regulation. This can lead to symptoms such as shakiness, sweating, irritability, and in severe cases, seizures. It is crucial to monitor and gradually adjust glucose intake in newborns on parenteral nutrition to prevent the occurrence of reactive hypoglycemia and maintain stable blood sugar levels.

Question 152:

Correct Answer: B) Administration or extraction of a peripherally inserted central catheter (PICC line).

Explanation: Insertion or removal of a peripherally inserted central catheter (PICC line) is a common procedure in neonatal care that may require the use of an opioid to alleviate pain. This procedure involves the placement or removal of a long, thin tube into a major vein, usually in the arm or leg, to provide medication or fluids directly into the bloodstream. Infants undergoing this procedure may experience discomfort, anxiety, or pain due to the manipulation of their delicate veins. The use of an opioid, such as morphine or fentanyl, can be deemed suitable in this scenario to help alleviate pain and minimize distress for the neonate. Opioids are potent analgesics that work by binding to specific receptors in the brain and spinal cord, blocking pain signals and inducing a sense of relaxation. The administration of opioids in neonatal care is carefully monitored by medical professionals to ensure appropriate dosing and minimize potential side effects. By utilizing opioids during the insertion or removal of a PICC line, healthcare providers can prioritize the comfort and well-being of the neonate, ultimately ensuring a smoother and less painful procedure.

Question 153:

Correct Answer: C) Hypoplastic left heart syndrome

Explanation: Hypoplastic left heart syndrome is a type of congenital heart disease that leads to cyanosis. It occurs when the left side of the heart, including the left ventricle and aortic valve, is underdeveloped. This condition obstructs blood flow from the heart to the body, causing oxygen-poor blood to mix with oxygen-rich blood. As a result, cyanosis, a bluish discoloration of the skin, lips, and nails due to inadequate oxygen supply, becomes apparent. Infants born with hypoplastic left heart syndrome often experience difficulty breathing, fatigue, and poor feeding. Immediate medical intervention, including surgery, is typically required to correct this life-threatening condition and improve the child's overall prognosis.

Question 154:

Correct Answer: A) Meconium aspiration syndrome

Explanation: Meconium aspiration syndrome is the most probable diagnosis for the symptoms described in the case of the newborn baby. This condition occurs when a baby inhales meconium, which is the baby's first feces, into the lungs during or before delivery. The aspiration of meconium can cause airway obstruction and inflammation, leading to respiratory distress. The retractions during breathing and the grunting noise accompanying fast breaths are classic signs of respiratory distress in newborns with meconium aspiration syndrome. Prompt recognition and intervention are crucial to manage this condition and prevent further complications. Immediate medical attention and supportive care, such as oxygen therapy and mechanical ventilation if necessary, are typically required to improve the baby's respiratory function and overall well-being.

Question 155:

Correct Answer: B) An omphalocele is characterized by the protrusion of abdominal contents through the umbilicus, whereas in gastroschisis, the abdominal organs lack a protective membrane cover.

Explanation: An omphalocele occurs when the abdominal contents protrude through the umbilicus, but a gastroschisis occurs when there is no membrane covering the abdominal organs. This distinction is crucial in understanding the differences between the two conditions. In an omphalocele, there is a sac or covering present, which contains the herniated organs. This sac is formed by the peritoneum and the amniotic membrane. On the other hand, in gastroschisis, there is no protective sac, leaving the abdominal organs exposed directly to the amniotic fluid. This lack of membrane coverage makes gastroschisis more prone to complications such as infection and damage to the exposed organs. Therefore, distinguishing between an omphalocele and a gastroschisis is vital for accurate diagnosis and appropriate management of these conditions.

Question 156:

Correct Answer: B) Examine the infant's entire body for signs of cyanosis in the extremities and check for retractions or other indications of respiratory distress.

Explanation: Assess the rest of the newborn's body to determine the presence of cyanosis in the extremities or any signs of respiratory distress such as retractions. This initial course of action is crucial as it helps the nurse gather more information about the overall condition of the baby. If cyanosis is present in the extremities or if the infant is displaying signs of respiratory distress, immediate medical intervention may be required. On the other hand, if there are no additional concerning signs, further assessment can be conducted to identify the cause of the bluish discoloration around the mouth. By prioritizing the assessment of the baby's body, the nurse can ensure a timely and appropriate response to the observed symptoms.

Question 157:

Correct Answer: C) Trisomy 21

Explanation: Trisomy 21, commonly known as Down syndrome, is typically indicated when a quad screen test reveals specific abnormal levels. This condition is characterized by an extra copy of chromosome 21, resulting in developmental and intellectual disabilities. The decreased levels of AFP, elevated hCG, reduced uE_3, and increased INH-A observed in the quad-screen test are indicative of Trisomy 21. These biomarkers provide valuable information about the fetus's overall health and the likelihood of Down syndrome. It is important to note that further diagnostic testing, such as amniocentesis or chorionic villus sampling, is usually recommended to confirm the diagnosis and provide more accurate information for making informed decisions.

Question 158:

Correct Answer: A) 60% to 70%

Explanation: The proportion of cerebrospinal glucose level in comparison to the plasma glucose level should ideally be around 60% to 70%. This range is considered optimal for maintaining normal brain function and providing energy to the central nervous system. The brain relies heavily on glucose as its primary source of fuel, and maintaining a consistent supply is crucial for its proper functioning. Deviations from this range can indicate underlying health conditions such as infections or metabolic disorders. Therefore, it is important to ensure that the cerebrospinal glucose level remains within this proportion to support optimal brain health and function.

Question 159:

Correct Answer: C) Cerebral palsy

Explanation: Periventricular leukomalacia (PVL) is a condition characterized by damage to the white matter of the brain, particularly around the ventricles. This damage occurs primarily in preterm infants due to factors such as oxygen deprivation and inflammation. While the severity and outcomes of PVL can vary, one of the most common conditions that these newborns are more likely to develop is cerebral palsy. Cerebral palsy is a group of motor disorders that affect muscle control and coordination, resulting in physical disabilities. The damage to the white matter in PVL can disrupt the normal development of the brain, leading to motor impairments often seen in cerebral palsy. Therefore, it is important to closely monitor and provide appropriate interventions for newborns with PVL to manage the potential development of cerebral palsy.

Question 160:

Correct Answer: B) The baby is experiencing CPAP failure

Explanation: CPAP failure is indicated when a newborn baby, who arrived prematurely at 31 weeks and exhibited symptoms of respiratory distress syndrome, requires a FiO2 of 0.40 shortly after being placed on CPAP post-birth. CPAP, or continuous positive airway pressure, is a non-invasive ventilation method used to support the baby's breathing by delivering a constant flow of air and keeping the airways open. However, if the baby's condition worsens and a higher FiO2 is needed to maintain adequate oxygen levels, it suggests that CPAP alone is not effectively managing respiratory distress. This highlights the failure of CPAP as the primary treatment, indicating the need for further intervention or a different respiratory support strategy.

Question 161:

Correct Answer: C) A premature infant being formula fed

Explanation: Necrotizing enterocolitis (NEC) is a serious gastrointestinal disease that primarily affects premature infants. Among them, those who are formula-fed are at the highest risk of contracting this condition. A premature infant being formula fed is more vulnerable to NEC due to several factors. Firstly, premature babies have an underdeveloped immune system and immature digestive tract, making them more susceptible to infections and inflammation. Secondly, formula feeding can introduce harmful bacteria and disrupt the delicate balance of gut flora, further increasing the risk of NEC. Additionally, breast milk contains numerous protective factors that help prevent NEC, which are absent in formula milk. Therefore, it is crucial to prioritize breastfeeding or provide pasteurized donor breast milk to premature infants to minimize the risk of NEC.

Question 162:

Correct Answer: B) First

Explanation: First, it is important to understand that the susceptibility of an unborn baby to developing birth defects when the mother contracts toxoplasmosis can vary depending on the stage of pregnancy. However, during the first trimester, the unborn baby is most vulnerable to the harmful effects of toxoplasmosis infection. This is because the first trimester is a critical period of organ development and differentiation. If the infection occurs during this time, it can significantly impact the formation and function of vital organs, leading to severe birth defects. Therefore, it is crucial for pregnant women to take precautions to prevent toxoplasmosis infection, especially during the first trimester, to safeguard the health and development of their unborn baby.

Question 163:

Correct Answer: A) 60 minutes

Explanation: Within 60 minutes after delivery, it is highly recommended that neonates with a very low birth weight (VLBW) initiate skin-to-skin contact, also known as kangaroo care, with their mother. This immediate bonding and physical closeness between the mother and the baby have shown numerous benefits for both the newborn and the mother. By starting kangaroo care within this timeframe, the neonate experiences several advantages, such as improved temperature regulation, stable heart and respiratory rates, enhanced breastfeeding initiation, and reduced stress levels. It also promotes the development of a secure and nurturing attachment between the mother and the baby, which is crucial for their long-term emotional well-being. Therefore, initiating skin-to-skin contact within 60 minutes after delivery is vital for the optimal health and development of neonates with a very low birth weight.

Question 164:

Correct Answer: A) Try a tube that is a half size smaller

Explanation: In the scenario where a new tracheostomy tube cannot be successfully inserted into a newborn after two attempts, the subsequent course of action should be to try a tube that is a half size smaller. This approach is recommended due to the possibility that the initial attempts might have been hindered by the chosen tube size being too large for the newborn's anatomy. By opting for a smaller tube size, it allows for a better fit and increased chances of successful insertion. It is crucial to consider the importance of appropriate tube sizing for the newborn's comfort, optimal ventilation, and prevention of complications. Therefore, trying a tube that is a half size smaller is a logical and practical solution in such a situation.

Question 165:

Correct Answer: C) Toxoplasmosis

Explanation: Toxoplasmosis is a parasitic infection that can potentially be caused by the excrement of domestic felines. This disease is caused by the Toxoplasma gondii parasite, which primarily infects warm-blooded animals, including humans. The parasite can be found in the feces of infected cats, and it can contaminate soil, water, and various other surfaces. Humans can become infected by inadvertently ingesting the parasite through contaminated food or water, or by directly handling cat litter or soil contaminated with cat feces. While most healthy individuals experience mild flu-like symptoms or no symptoms at all, toxoplasmosis can pose serious risks to individuals with weakened immune systems or pregnant women, as it can cause severe complications. Therefore, it is crucial to handle cat litter and soil with caution and maintain good hygiene practices to prevent toxoplasmosis infection.

Question 166:

Correct Answer: C) 80%

Explanation: 80% of the iron from breast milk would be absorbed by the infant's body. This high absorption rate can be attributed to the fact that breast milk naturally contains bioavailable iron, which is easily absorbed by the infant's digestive system. On the other hand, formula iron is often added in a less absorbable form, resulting in only about a tenth of it being absorbed. Breast milk is not only rich in iron, but it also contains other components that enhance iron absorption, such as lactoferrin and vitamin C. These factors contribute to the higher proportion of iron absorption from breast milk compared to formula.

Question 167:

Correct Answer: B) 20 mL per aliquot

Explanation: In the scenario described, the newborn baby with isoimmune hemolytic anemia requires an exchange transfusion. During this procedure, the baby's blood is gradually replaced with donor blood to remove the affected blood cells. To ensure a safe and effective exchange, it is crucial to determine the appropriate volume for each aliquot that needs to be taken out and replaced. In this case, the recommended volume for each aliquot is 20 mL. This volume is carefully calculated based on the baby's weight and the desired reduction in the affected blood cells. By removing and replacing 20 mL of blood at a time, the exchange transfusion can be performed in a controlled manner while minimizing any potential risks or complications.

Question 168:

Correct Answer: B) Heart failure

Explanation: Heart failure is the primary reason behind the occurrence of central cyanosis. When the heart fails to pump blood effectively, it can lead to inadequate oxygen delivery to the body's tissues. As a result, the oxygen saturation in the blood decreases, leading to cyanosis. Central cyanosis specifically refers to the bluish discoloration of the lips, tongue, and mucous membranes, indicating low levels of oxygen in arterial blood. Heart failure can occur due to various factors such as coronary artery disease, heart valve disorders, or cardiomyopathy. Prompt medical intervention is crucial to diagnose and manage heart failure, as it can significantly impact an individual's overall health and quality of life.

Question 169:

Correct Answer: C) Engaging in play activities with the baby

Explanation: Playing with the infant is a method of providing care that incorporates socioemotional aspects. This approach recognizes the importance of nurturing a child's emotional well-being in addition to meeting their physical needs. By engaging in play, caregivers can establish a bond with the infant, promote emotional development, and enhance their social skills. Play also allows infants to express their emotions, explore their environment, and develop their cognitive abilities. Furthermore, playing with the infant can create a safe and secure environment, fostering trust and attachment. Overall, incorporating socioemotional elements through play is vital for the holistic care and development of an infant.

Question 170:

Correct Answer: B) Vitamin D

Explanation: Vitamin D is typically required as a supplement for infants who are being breastfed. Breast milk is an excellent source of nutrients for babies, but it may not provide adequate amounts of vitamin D. Vitamin D is crucial for the proper development and growth of infants, as it plays a vital role in bone health and immune function. Since breast milk is low in vitamin D, supplementation is recommended to ensure that infants receive the necessary amount. Vitamin D supplementation is particularly important for infants who are exclusively breastfed, as they may not receive enough sunlight exposure, which is a natural source of vitamin D. Therefore, providing infants with a vitamin D supplement is essential to support their overall health and well-being.

Question 171:

Correct Answer: C) Early feedings

Explanation: Early feedings are the recommended preventive measure for newborns, including baby Michael, who are susceptible to low blood sugar levels. This approach entails initiating feedings soon after birth, typically within the first hour. Early feedings help provide newborns with the necessary nutrients, including glucose, to stabilize their blood sugar levels. By ensuring regular and frequent feedings, the baby's body can maintain a steady supply of glucose, reducing the risk of hypoglycemia. Additionally, early feedings also promote bonding between the newborn and the caregiver, stimulate the baby's digestive system, and support overall growth and development. Hence, early feedings serve as an effective preventive measure against low blood sugar levels in susceptible newborns like baby Michael.

Question 172:

Correct Answer: C) Hirschsprung's disease

Explanation: Hirschsprung's disease is a potential health issue that the newborn baby in the Neonatal Intensive Care Unit could be facing. This condition is characterized by the absence of nerve cells in certain parts of the baby's colon, leading to an inability to pass stool. The lack of bowel movement in the initial 48 hours after birth and the presence of vomiting during oral feeding attempts are indicative of this condition. Hirschsprung's disease can cause a blockage in the baby's intestines, leading to the accumulation of stool and subsequent vomiting. Early diagnosis and intervention are crucial to prevent complications and ensure the baby's well-being.

Question 173:

Correct Answer: B) Hypoglycemia

Explanation: Hypoglycemia is a condition that a hypothermic newborn is more likely to develop. When a newborn is hypothermic, their body temperature drops significantly, leading to a decrease in metabolic processes. This decrease in metabolism can affect the regulation of blood sugar levels, causing hypoglycemia. Hypoglycemia occurs when the blood glucose levels drop below normal, and it can have severe consequences for a newborn, such as impaired brain function and developmental delays. Therefore, it is crucial to closely monitor hypothermic newborns for signs of hypoglycemia and provide prompt intervention to prevent any potential complications.

Question 174:

Correct Answer: A) Adhesive

Explanation: Adhesive is the primary reason for skin deterioration in newborn babies. The use of medical adhesives, such as tapes and bandages, can cause damage to their delicate skin. Adhesives have the potential to strip away the top layer of the skin, leading to redness, irritation, and even blistering. The sensitive skin of newborns is more prone to such damage as it is thinner and has a less developed protective barrier. Furthermore, prolonged exposure to adhesives can disrupt the natural moisture balance of the skin, causing dryness and further exacerbating skin deterioration. Therefore, it is crucial to handle newborns' skin with utmost care and choose appropriate alternatives to minimize the risk of adhesive-related skin problems.

Question 175:

Correct Answer: A) Compensated respiratory acidosis

Explanation: Compensated respiratory acidosis occurs when the body attempts to restore the pH balance in the blood in response to high levels of carbon dioxide (pCO2). In this case, the newborn baby's arterial blood gas values indicate a pH of 7.36, pCO2 of 52, and HCO3 (bicarbonate) of 30. These values suggest that the baby is experiencing compensated respiratory acidosis. Compensated respiratory acidosis is characterized by an increased pCO2, indicating an inability to effectively eliminate carbon dioxide through respiration. The body compensates for this by retaining more bicarbonate (HCO3), which increases the overall pH level, preventing it from dropping to acidic levels. Therefore, although the baby's blood gas values indicate an imbalance, the body's compensatory mechanisms have successfully maintained the pH within a normal range.

Question 176:

Correct Answer: C) 25%

Explanation: 25% is the likelihood of a newborn developing sickle cell disease if both parents are carriers of the sickle cell trait. Sickle cell disease is an autosomal recessive condition, meaning that for the child to develop the disease, they must inherit two copies of the abnormal gene, one from each parent. In this scenario, there are four possible combinations of genes that the child can inherit: two normal genes, one normal and one abnormal gene, one abnormal and one normal gene, or two abnormal genes. With a 25% probability, there is a one in four chance that the child will inherit two abnormal genes and develop sickle cell disease. It is important for parents who are carriers to be aware of this risk and seek genetic counseling to make informed decisions about family planning.

Question 177:

Correct Answer: C) Down syndrome

Explanation: Down syndrome is a genetic disorder commonly associated with atrioventricular septal defect (AVSD) or, in milder cases, ventricular septal defect (VSD), which a neonatal intensive care nurse might encounter. Down syndrome, also known as trisomy 21, is caused by the presence of an extra copy of chromosome 21. This additional genetic material affects the development of various organs and systems in the body, including the heart. AVSD and VSD are two common heart defects observed in individuals with Down syndrome. AVSD occurs when there is a hole in the center of the heart, affecting the septum and the valves. VSD, on the other hand, is a defect in the septum that separates the heart's ventricles. The presence of these heart defects in neonates with Down syndrome necessitates specialized care and monitoring in the neonatal intensive care unit.

Question 178:

Correct Answer: C) Inform her that it's not permissible to divulge any information, however, you will notify the parents about her call and request them to get in touch with her.

Explanation: The most appropriate response from the nurse in this situation would be to inform the grandmother, "Tell her you are not able to give her any information, but that you will let the parents know she called and ask them to contact her." It is crucial for the nurse to prioritize patient confidentiality and privacy. By not disclosing any information about Timmy's health status over the phone, the nurse upholds ethical standards and ensures that the patient's privacy is protected. However, the nurse shows empathy and concern for the grandmother by promising to relay her message to the parents and request them to contact her. This approach maintains professionalism while acknowledging the grandmother's need for an update and providing a means of communication between her and Timmy's parents.

Question 179:

Correct Answer: B) Lower

Explanation: Lower PaCO2 levels in the venous umbilical cord blood compared to the arterial umbilical cord blood can be attributed to several physiological factors. Firstly, the venous blood in the umbilical cord carries deoxygenated blood from the fetus back to the placenta. This blood has already delivered oxygen and nutrients to the fetal tissues, resulting in a lower concentration of carbon dioxide. Additionally, the umbilical vein transports blood that bypasses the fetal lungs, leading to a decrease in the levels of carbon dioxide. Therefore, it is expected that the PaCO2 level in the venous umbilical cord blood would be lower than that in the arterial umbilical cord blood.

Question 180:

Correct Answer: A) 3 to 4 days

Explanation: In the Neonatal Intensive Care Unit (NICU), it is recommended to exclusively feed newborns with colostrum for a period of 3 to 4 days. This initial milk produced by the mother is rich in antibodies and essential nutrients that provide numerous health benefits to the newborn. Colostrum helps in boosting the baby's immune system, protecting against infections, and aiding in the development of the gastrointestinal tract. Additionally, colostrum acts as a natural laxative, helping the baby pass meconium (the first stool) and preventing jaundice. By exclusively feeding newborns with colostrum for 3 to 4 days, healthcare providers ensure that the baby receives the maximum benefits from this vital source of nutrition and immune protection.

Question 181:

Correct Answer: C) Provide a pacifier dipped in sucrose for 2 minutes before the heel lance

Explanation: To mitigate discomfort when collecting a capillary blood sample by piercing a newborn's heel, providing a pacifier dipped in sucrose for 2 minutes before the heel lance is the best approach. This method has been proven effective in reducing pain and distress during medical procedures in infants. The use of a pacifier provides non-nutritive sucking, which has a soothing effect on newborns by stimulating the release of endorphins, natural pain-relieving substances in the body. Additionally, sucrose, a sweet-tasting solution, has been shown to have analgesic properties and can further alleviate pain and discomfort. By combining these two approaches, healthcare professionals can help minimize the stress and pain experienced by newborns during capillary blood sampling, ultimately leading to a more positive and comfortable experience for both the baby and their caregiver.

Question 182:

Correct Answer: A) Apply warm saline-soaked gauze and plastic wrap over the exposed tissue

Explanation: In the scenario of a newborn baby with a significant myelomeningocele, the first course of action should be to apply warm saline-soaked gauze and plastic wrap over the exposed tissue. This immediate intervention is crucial to provide a sterile environment, prevent infection, and protect the delicate neural tissue. By applying warm saline-soaked gauze, the wound can be gently cleansed and any debris or bacteria can be removed. The plastic wrap acts as a barrier, shielding the exposed tissue from further contamination and reducing the risk of complications. This initial step is essential in the management of myelomeningocele and sets the foundation for subsequent surgical repair and ongoing care.

Question 183:

Correct Answer: A) Right ventricle

Explanation: The right ventricle is the part of the heart that would be most impacted if pulmonary stenosis is left untreated. Pulmonary stenosis is a condition characterized by the narrowing of the pulmonary valve, which is responsible for regulating blood flow from the right ventricle to the lungs. When this valve is constricted, the right ventricle has to work harder to pump blood through the narrowed opening. Over time, this increased workload can lead to the thickening and enlargement of the right ventricle, causing it to become weaker and less efficient. Consequently, the right ventricle may struggle to pump blood effectively, resulting in various complications and symptoms associated with untreated pulmonary stenosis.

Question 184:

Correct Answer: C) Lactation consults

Explanation: Lactation consult is a crucial topic to incorporate into the discharge planning and education for this premature baby girl. As she has been doing well with bottle feedings and has successfully nursed twice, it is evident that breastfeeding is a viable option for her. However, premature babies often face unique challenges when it comes to breastfeeding, such as latching difficulties and insufficient milk supply. Therefore, involving a lactation consultant in the discharge planning is essential to provide the necessary support and guidance to the mother. The lactation consultant can provide education on proper breastfeeding techniques, help with establishing a good latch, and offer guidance on increasing milk supply if needed. Their expertise will ensure that the transition to breastfeeding at home is successful and beneficial for both the baby and the mother.

Question 185:

Correct Answer: C) Only female newborns are affected

Explanation: Turner's syndrome is a genetic disorder that predominantly affects females only. This condition occurs when one of the X chromosomes is partially or completely missing in a female's cells. Typically, females have two X chromosomes (XX), while males have one X and one Y chromosome (XY). However, in individuals with Turner's syndrome, there is a missing or abnormal X chromosome, leading to a range of physical and developmental abnormalities. These can include short stature, infertility, heart defects, and learning difficulties. Due to the absence or alteration of the X chromosome, Turner's syndrome does not occur in newborn boys, making it exclusive to females.

Question 186:

Correct Answer: C) Human breast milk is deficient in protein content.

Explanation: Breast milk contains insufficient protein, which is the main reason for adding breast milk fortifiers to the human breast milk given to premature newborns. Premature infants have higher protein requirements compared to full-term babies due to their rapid growth and development needs. Breast milk alone may not provide enough protein to support their nutritional needs, leading to potential growth and development deficits. By adding breast milk fortifiers, which are specially formulated to increase the protein content, premature infants receive the necessary nutrients to support their growth and development. These fortifiers help bridge the gap between the protein content in breast milk and the requirements of premature infants, ensuring optimal nutrition for their overall well-being.

Question 187:

Correct Answer: A) The right shoulder and lower abdomen

Explanation: The right shoulder and lower abdomen are the ideal locations for placing electrodes to monitor transcutaneous carbon dioxide (TCO2) levels in newborns like baby James suspected of having a right-to-left shunt due to an open ductus arteriosus. Placing the electrodes in these specific areas allows for accurate and reliable TCO2 measurements. The right shoulder placement ensures proper electrode contact with the skin, while the lower abdomen placement ensures minimal interference and optimal signal transmission. Monitoring TCO2 levels in these locations enables healthcare professionals to assess the effectiveness of treatment interventions, evaluate respiratory status, and ensure appropriate management of the right-to-left shunt.

Question 188:

Correct Answer: B) It reduces the osmotic concentration of formulas.

Explanation: The purpose of replacing lactose with glucose polymers in infant feedings is to lower the osmotic concentration of formulas. This is advantageous because it ensures that the formula is more easily digested by infants. Lactose, which is the natural sugar found in breast milk, can sometimes be difficult for infants to break down, leading to discomfort and digestive issues. By using glucose polymers instead, the osmotic concentration of the formula is reduced, making it easier for the baby's immature digestive system to handle. This substitution allows for better absorption and utilization of nutrients, promoting healthy growth and development in infants.

Question 189:

Correct Answer: B) The foreskin has to be completely retracted for cleaning and Dry the area well

Explanation: The foreskin should be completely retracted for cleaning and the area should be dried well. This is an important aspect of care for newborn baby boys who have not been circumcised. It is essential to ensure proper hygiene to prevent any potential infections or discomfort. When cleaning the area, parents should gently retract the foreskin and clean it with water and mild soap. It is important to avoid using harsh soaps or lotions that may irritate the delicate skin. After cleaning, the area should be thoroughly dried to prevent any moisture buildup which can lead to irritation or infection. By following these care guidelines, parents can ensure the well-being and comfort of their newborn son.

Question 190:

Correct Answer: A) Fentanyl

Explanation: Fentanyl is the medication most likely to be involved in significant drug-to-drug interactions (DDIs) in newborns. This potent opioid analgesic is commonly used for pain management in neonatal intensive care units. Fentanyl undergoes extensive metabolism in the liver, primarily mediated by the enzyme cytochrome P450 3A4 (CYP3A4). As a result, it interacts with other medications that are also metabolized by CYP3A4, leading to potential DDIs. Examples of drugs that can interact with fentanyl include antifungals (such as fluconazole), macrolide antibiotics (like erythromycin), and protease inhibitors (such as ritonavir). These interactions can result in altered fentanyl metabolism, leading to potential toxicity or reduced efficacy. Therefore, healthcare providers must exercise caution when administering fentanyl to newborns, considering the potential for significant DDIs.

Question 191:

Correct Answer: C) 5 minutes attempt at sucking a fully pumped breast

Explanation: Transitioning neonates who are 34 weeks or older and require nasal continuous positive airway pressure (CPAP) to breastfeeding should include an initial attempt of 5 minutes at sucking a fully pumped breast. This approach is crucial in promoting successful breastfeeding in this population. By allowing the neonate to engage in sucking, they can practice the necessary skills required for effective breastfeeding. Encouraging a 5-minute attempt ensures that the neonate has sufficient time to establish a latch and initiate milk transfer. Furthermore, starting with a fully pumped breast provides a consistent and reliable milk flow, facilitating the neonate's ability to coordinate sucking, swallowing, and breathing. This approach aids in the development of proper feeding techniques and increases the likelihood of successful breastfeeding initiation.

Question 192:

Correct Answer: A) DiGeorge syndrome

Explanation: DiGeorge syndrome is a condition associated with a chromosomal abnormality in chromosome 22. This genetic disorder occurs when a small piece of chromosome 22 is deleted during the early development of an individual. DiGeorge syndrome is characterized by a wide range of symptoms, including heart defects, immune system abnormalities, and facial abnormalities. These symptoms can vary significantly from person to person, making diagnosis challenging. The chromosomal abnormality in chromosome 22 disrupts the development of several organs and systems in the body, leading to the diverse features of DiGeorge syndrome. Early detection and intervention are crucial in managing the condition and providing appropriate medical care and support for individuals with DiGeorge syndrome.

Question 193:

Correct Answer: C) Supraventricular tachycardia

Explanation: Supraventricular tachycardia (SVT) is a condition that can be suggested by the pattern observed in a newborn's ECG tracing. SVT is characterized by a rapid heart rate originating from the upper chambers of the heart, known as the atria. In an ECG tracing, SVT may be indicated by a consistent and abnormal heart rate above 220 beats per minute in newborns. This pattern is distinct from the normal sinus rhythm seen in a healthy newborn's ECG tracing. SVT can pose risks to newborns, including inadequate blood flow and oxygenation. Therefore, prompt diagnosis and management are crucial to prevent complications and ensure the well-being of the newborn.

Question 194:

Correct Answer: A) An initial high dose

Explanation: A loading dose is typically necessary for a newborn baby to quickly achieve a steady state of a medication's plasma concentration. This approach involves administering a higher initial dose of the medication to rapidly reach the desired therapeutic level in the bloodstream. Since newborns have a smaller blood volume and a faster metabolism compared to adults, a loading dose helps overcome these factors to achieve the desired therapeutic effect more rapidly. This is particularly important for medications that require a steady state for optimal efficacy, such as antibiotics or anticonvulsants. By administering a loading dose, healthcare professionals can ensure that the newborn receives an adequate amount of the medication from the start, expediting the attainment of a stable plasma concentration.

Question 195:

Correct Answer: B) 5 to 7 weeks

Explanation: At around 5 to 7 weeks, the breast milk of a preterm baby begins to exhibit similar characteristics as that of a full-term baby. During this period, the composition of breast milk gradually changes to meet the unique nutritional needs of preterm infants. Initially, the milk produced by mothers of preterm babies is different from that of full-term babies, as it contains higher levels of protein, fat, and other essential nutrients. However, as the baby grows and their digestive system develops, the breast milk gradually adjusts its composition to match the nutritional content found in the breast milk of full-term babies. This transition allows preterm babies to receive optimal nutrition and support their growth and development.

Question 196:

Correct Answer: C) Initiation of fluid replenishment is necessary.

Explanation: Fluid replacement is indicated when the discharge from a newly formed colostomy is measured at 4 mL/kg/hour. This measurement indicates a significant amount of fluid loss, which can lead to dehydration and electrolyte imbalances. Fluid replacement is necessary to restore the body's fluid balance and prevent complications. By providing additional fluids, the body can maintain proper hydration, support vital organ functions, and promote healing. It is essential to monitor the patient's fluid intake and output closely to ensure adequate replacement. Prompt intervention and appropriate fluid management are crucial in preventing further complications and promoting optimal recovery.

Question 197:

Correct Answer: A) 60 bpm

Explanation: In the context of neonatal resuscitation, the heart rate threshold at which a neonate should begin to receive chest compressions, assuming they are already receiving sufficient and effective ventilation, is 60 bpm. At this point, it is crucial to provide cardiac massage to further support the circulation of the newborn. Chest compressions help to maintain an adequate blood flow and oxygen delivery to vital organs, which is essential for the neonate's survival. By initiating chest compressions at a heart rate of 60 bpm, healthcare professionals can effectively intervene and increase the chances of a successful resuscitation.

Question 198:

Correct Answer: B) Thrombocytopenia

Explanation: Renal vein thrombosis in newborns is often associated with various clinical signs, with thrombocytopenia being a key indicator. Thrombocytopenia refers to a condition characterized by abnormally low levels of platelets in the blood. In the context of renal vein thrombosis, the underlying thrombus formation can impede blood flow and disrupt normal platelet function. Consequently, thrombocytopenia can manifest as excessive bleeding, easy bruising, or petechiae, which are small red or purple spots on the skin. Additionally, reduced platelet count can contribute to impaired clotting, leading to prolonged bleeding episodes. Therefore, thrombocytopenia serves as an important clinical sign in diagnosing renal vein thrombosis in newborns.

Question 199:

Correct Answer: C) Benzathine penicillin, one 2.4-million-unit injection

Explanation: Benzathine penicillin, one 2.4-million-unit injection, is the preferred method of treatment for a pregnant woman diagnosed with primary syphilis. This antibiotic is highly effective in treating syphilis and has been the standard treatment for many years. It is the recommended treatment by the Centers for Disease Control and Prevention (CDC) and other medical organizations. Syphilis can have serious consequences for both the pregnant woman and her unborn baby. If left untreated, it can lead to complications such as stillbirth, preterm delivery, or congenital syphilis in the infant. Therefore, it is crucial to initiate treatment as soon as possible to prevent these potential adverse outcomes. Benzathine penicillin is the drug of choice for treating syphilis in pregnancy due to its ability to reach therapeutic levels in the bloodstream for an extended period. A single injection of 2.4 million units provides adequate treatment for primary syphilis, ensuring that the infection is eradicated. It is important to note that alternative treatments, such as oral antibiotics, are not recommended for pregnant women with syphilis. These alternatives may not be as effective in clearing the infection and preventing complications. Therefore, benzathine penicillin remains the preferred method of treatment for pregnant women diagnosed with primary syphilis.

Question 200:

Correct Answer: B) Cephalohematoma

Explanation: Cephalohematoma is a significant risk factor that can lead to the development of severe hyperbilirubinemia. It is a condition characterized by the accumulation of blood between the skull bone and the tough outer covering of the brain. When a cephalohematoma occurs, there is a risk of increased breakdown of red blood cells, resulting in the release of bilirubin. Bilirubin is a yellow pigment that is produced during the normal breakdown of red blood cells. However, when there is an excessive accumulation of bilirubin in the body, it can lead to severe hyperbilirubinemia. This condition can cause jaundice, which is characterized by yellowing of the skin and eyes. Therefore, cephalohematoma poses a significant risk for the development of severe hyperbilirubinemia.

Question 201:

Correct Answer: B) Pain relief

Explanation: Pain relief is the primary purpose of administering oral sucrose to newborns. Sucrose, a natural sugar, has been widely used as an effective analgesic in neonatal care. By activating the sweet taste receptors on the tongue, sucrose triggers the release of endogenous opioids, which are natural pain-relieving substances in the body. This mechanism helps to alleviate pain and discomfort during various medical procedures, such as blood sampling, heel sticks, or immunizations. Additionally, sucrose administration has been found to have calming and soothing effects on newborns, promoting relaxation and reducing stress. Overall, the use of oral sucrose is a safe and non-invasive method to provide pain relief to newborns, enhancing their comfort and well-being during medical interventions.

Question 202:

Correct Answer: A) Full-term infants

Explanation: Full-term infants are more frequently observed to experience hypoxic ischemic encephalopathy. This condition occurs when there is a lack of oxygen and blood flow to the brain, leading to potential brain damage. The risk of hypoxic ischemic encephalopathy is higher in full-term infants due to various factors. Firstly, full-term infants have a more developed central nervous system compared to preterm infants, making them more susceptible to brain injury from oxygen deprivation. Additionally, complications during labor and delivery, such as umbilical cord compression or placental abruption, can occur more commonly in full-term infants, further increasing the likelihood of hypoxic ischemic encephalopathy. Therefore, it is important to closely monitor and provide appropriate care to full-term infants to mitigate the risk of this condition.

Question 203:

Correct Answer: B) Administering pain medication to a patient prior to conducting wound care.

Explanation: Waiting until a patient has had pain medication before performing wound care is a clear example of nonmaleficence in nursing. Nonmaleficence is an ethical principle that emphasizes the duty to do no harm to the patient. In this instance, the nurse is prioritizing the patient's comfort and well-being by ensuring they are adequately medicated to manage their pain before initiating a potentially painful procedure such as wound care. By waiting for the pain medication to take effect, the nurse is minimizing the potential harm and discomfort that the patient may experience during wound care. This approach aligns with the fundamental principle of nonmaleficence, demonstrating a commitment to promoting the patient's overall health and avoiding unnecessary suffering.

Question 204:

Correct Answer: B) A contrast enema

Explanation: A contrast enema is the preferred initial diagnostic procedure when a newborn, like baby Charles, is suspected to have a lower bowel obstruction. This procedure involves introducing a contrast material, usually barium or a water-soluble contrast, into the rectum to visualize the lower gastrointestinal tract and identify any potential obstructions. A contrast enema provides valuable information regarding the location, extent, and nature of the obstruction, allowing healthcare professionals to make an accurate diagnosis and determine the most appropriate course of treatment. By highlighting any structural abnormalities or blockages in the lower bowel, a contrast enema effectively assists in guiding further management decisions, such as surgery or conservative management, ensuring the best possible outcome for the newborn.

Question 205:

Correct Answer: C) Hydrops fetalis

Explanation: Hydrops fetalis is a medical condition that can occur in a newborn baby due to Rh factor incompatibility. This condition is characterized by an abnormal accumulation of fluid in two or more fetal compartments. It is caused by the destruction of red blood cells in the fetus as a result of Rh incompatibility between the mother and baby's blood types. When a mother is Rh-negative and the baby is Rh-positive, the mother's immune system can produce antibodies that attack the baby's red blood cells. This leads to severe anemia and fluid buildup in the fetus, affecting various organs and systems. If left untreated, hydrops fetalis can be life-threatening for the newborn baby. Early diagnosis and proper management are crucial to improve the chances of a positive outcome.

Question 206:

Correct Answer: B) To confirm the comprehensive understanding of imparted information.

Explanation: To ensure that the information that is taught is fully understood, healthcare professionals often employ the Teach-Back method when providing education to patients and their families. This approach is a significant benefit as it promotes effective communication and comprehension. By encouraging patients to explain the information they have received in their own words, healthcare providers can gauge their understanding and identify any misconceptions. The Teach-Back method also allows patients and their families to actively participate in their own healthcare, promoting a sense of empowerment and engagement. This approach not only improves patient satisfaction but also enhances adherence to treatment plans and ultimately leads to better health outcomes. It is an invaluable tool in healthcare education that fosters comprehensive understanding and patient-centered care.

Question 207:

Correct Answer: B) A pregnant woman of 29 years, at her 26th week of gestation, experiencing abdominal discomfort after tumbling down a long staircase.

Explanation: The KleihauerBetke test would be beneficial in the situation of a 29-year-old pregnant female at 26 weeks gestation experiencing abdominal pain following a fall down a steep flight of stairs. This test is used to determine the extent of fetal-maternal hemorrhage (FMH) in cases of trauma or other conditions that may cause bleeding during pregnancy. FMH can occur when there is a disruption in the placenta or uterine wall, leading to the mixing of fetal and maternal blood. By quantifying the amount of fetal blood that has entered the maternal circulation, the KleihauerBetke test helps healthcare professionals assess the risk of fetalanemia and determine the need for further intervention, such as Rh immunoglobulin administration or fetal blood transfusion.

Question 208:

Correct Answer: B) Stimulate the neonate's back and limbs.

Explanation: To stimulate breathing in a newborn as part of the ABCs of neonatal resuscitation, the nurse should rub the neonate's back and extremities. This action is crucial in initiating the breathing process by providing tactile stimulation. Rubbing the back and extremities helps to awaken the baby's respiratory drive and encourages the initiation of spontaneous breaths. This technique promotes the activation of motor responses and reflexes, which are necessary for the newborn to take their first breaths. By stimulating the baby's sensory receptors through gentle rubbing, the nurse helps to establish a regular breathing pattern and ensures adequate oxygenation. Therefore, rubbing the neonate's back and extremities is an essential intervention to promote breathing and ensure the well-being of the newborn.

Question 209:

Correct Answer: C) Blood transfusion

Explanation: Blood transfusion is a critical neonatal intervention that requires the informed consent of a parent or legal guardian in emergency scenarios. This procedure involves the transfer of blood or blood components from a donor to a neonate who is in needs of blood replacement due to severe anemia, hemorrhage, or other life-threatening conditions. Informed consent is crucial as it ensures that parents or legal guardians fully understand the potential risks and benefits of the procedure, including the possibility of transfusion reactions, infections, or other complications. By obtaining informed consent, healthcare professionals can demonstrate respect for the autonomy and decision-making capacity of the parents or legal guardians, while also ensuring the best possible care for the neonate.

Question 210:

Correct Answer: B) Increased IWL by 40% to 50%

Explanation: Increased IWL by 40% to 50% is observed in newborns placed under radiant warmers in incubators compared to the standard IWL in neonates. This occurs due to the specific environment created by the radiant warmers. The heat generated by the radiant warmer increases the temperature around the newborn, leading to an increase in evaporation and subsequently, water loss. The radiant warmers create a drier environment, which enhances transepidermal water loss. This increase in IWL can have implications for the hydration status of the newborns, requiring close monitoring and appropriate fluid management. It is important for healthcare professionals to be aware of this difference in IWL to ensure adequate hydration and prevent any potential complications associated with excessive water loss.

Question 211:

Correct Answer: C) Newborn Transient Tachypnea

Explanation: Transient tachypnea of the newborn (TTN) is the primary reason for respiratory distress syndrome in a newborn. TTN occurs when there is an accumulation of fluid in the lungs, leading to difficulty in breathing. This condition typically occurs in full-term infants and is more common in babies born via cesarean section. The fluid in the lungs is usually cleared during the process of labor, but in some cases, it remains in the lungs, causing respiratory distress. TTN can lead to rapid breathing, grunting, flaring of the nostrils, and retractions. However, with appropriate medical intervention and support, the condition usually resolves within a few days.

Question 212:

Correct Answer: C) 5 to 7 mL

Explanation: On their first day of life, a newborn's stomach has an approximate capacity of 5 to 7 mL. This small size is due to the fact that newborns have tiny stomachs that are still developing and adjusting to the outside world. The small capacity ensures that the baby's digestive system is not overwhelmed and can handle the initial intake of breast milk or formula. As the baby grows and their digestive system matures, their stomach capacity will increase gradually. It is essential to understand and respect this limited capacity to avoid overfeeding and potential discomfort for the newborn.

Question 213:

Correct Answer: A) Proceed with a 5-10 cc warm water flush in the G-tube, and if resistance is encountered, perform aspiration and additional flushing."

Explanation: To address the issue of formula accumulation in the G-tube of the preterm baby in the Neonatal Intensive Care Unit (NICU), the nurse should take immediate action. The first step is to flush the tube with 5-10 cc of warm water. This will help to clear any blockage or obstruction that may be preventing the formula from flowing properly. Following this, the nurse should attempt to aspirate and flush the tube if there is resistance. This can help to further dislodge any potential blockage and ensure proper flow of the formula. By implementing these actions, the nurse can troubleshoot and resolve the problem effectively, ensuring that the baby receives the necessary nutrition without any complications.

Question 214:

Correct Answer: A) Caput succedaneum

Explanation: Caput succedaneum is the medical term used to describe the swelling of the head that extends beyond the suture lines in a newborn. This condition occurs as a result of the pressure exerted on the baby's skull during childbirth. The swelling usually appears shortly after delivery and is characterized by a soft, puffy mass on the scalp. While caput succedaneum may cause concern for parents, it is typically harmless and resolves on its own within a few days. It is important to differentiate caput succedaneum from other conditions like cephalohematoma, which involves bleeding beneath the skull and requires medical attention. By understanding the medical term for this swelling, healthcare professionals can accurately diagnose and reassure parents about their newborn's condition.

Question 215:

Correct Answer: C) 100 Â°F

Explanation: The standard temperature setting for both electric and disposable warming mattresses in neonatal care is 100 °F. This temperature is set to ensure that the infants' bodies are kept warm and maintained at a stable temperature. It is crucial to provide a controlled environment for newborns, especially those in neonatal care, as they are more susceptible to heat loss and hypothermia. By setting the temperature at 100 °F, healthcare professionals can effectively prevent heat loss and maintain the infants' body temperature within a safe range. This temperature setting is carefully determined based on extensive research and guidelines established by medical professionals, ensuring optimal care and comfort for neonates in their early stages of life.

Question 216:

Correct Answer: C) Infants with extremely low birth weight (below 1500 g)

Explanation: Very low birth weight infants (less than 1500 g) require the use of parenteral nutrition due to their vulnerable condition. Premature infants with such low birth weights often have underdeveloped digestive systems that are not yet capable of efficiently absorbing and processing nutrients from oral feedings. This can lead to inadequate growth and development, as well as potential complications such as malnutrition and growth failure. Parenteral nutrition, which involves delivering nutrients directly into the bloodstream through IV, ensures that these infants receive the essential macronutrients and micronutrients they need for optimal growth and development. By bypassing the immature digestive system, parenteral nutrition provides a reliable and controlled method of delivering essential nutrients to support the delicate health of very low birth weight infants.

Question 217:

Correct Answer: A) Hydrops fetalis

Explanation: Hydrops fetalis is a severe health complication that can arise in a newborn baby, such as baby Mia, due to Rh factor discrepancy. This condition occurs when the mother's Rh factor is negative and the baby's Rh factor is positive. When the baby's blood mixes with the mother's blood during pregnancy or delivery, the mother's immune system recognizes the baby's Rh-positive blood as a foreign substance and produces antibodies to attack it. These antibodies can cross the placenta and destroy the baby's red blood cells, leading to severe anemia and fluid buildup in various parts of the body. Hydrops fetalis can result in life-threatening complications, such as heart failure, respiratory distress, and organ failure. It requires immediate medical intervention, including blood transfusions and close monitoring, to improve the baby's chances of survival.

Question 218:

Correct Answer: B) Well-educated parents

Explanation: Well-educated parents are typically not a hurdle to the interaction between them and their newborn. This is because well-educated parents have access to information and resources that can help them understand and navigate the challenges of parenting. They are often more aware of the developmental needs of their newborn and can provide appropriate care and support. Additionally, their knowledge and understanding of child development may enhance their ability to effectively communicate and bond with their baby. Thus, well-educated parents are more likely to have the necessary skills and knowledge to establish a strong and nurturing relationship with their newborn, making them an asset rather than a hurdle in the parent-infant interaction.

Question 219:

Correct Answer: A) Within 1 hour of birth

Explanation: Within 1 hour of birth is the optimal time period for administering surfactant to a newborn baby experiencing respiratory distress. This early intervention is crucial as it helps improve lung function and prevents complications associated with respiratory distress syndrome (RDS). Administering surfactant within this timeframe aids in reducing the risk of respiratory failure, lung injury, and the need for more invasive interventions such as mechanical ventilation. By promptly administering surfactant, the baby's lungs can expand more easily, preventing the collapse of air sacs and facilitating the exchange of oxygen and carbon dioxide. This timely intervention significantly improves the baby's chances of a successful transition to breathing independently, ensuring better overall outcomes and reducing the risk of long-term complications.

Question 220:

Correct Answer: C) Four weeks postpartum

Explanation: Four weeks postpartum is the most common timeframe for the onset of postpartum depression. This refers to the period following childbirth when many women experience symptoms of depression. It is important to highlight that the majority of cases occur within this specific timeframe. Postpartum depression is a complex condition that can manifest in various ways, including feelings of sadness, anxiety, and fatigue. While some women may experience symptoms earlier or later than four weeks, it is crucial to be aware that this particular timeframe is the most prevalent. By acknowledging this, healthcare professionals can better identify and support women who may be at risk for postpartum depression during this critical period.

Question 221:

Correct Answer: B) Assisting patients in performing their ADLs when self-execution is not possible.

Explanation: Helping patients with their ADLs when they are not able to do them on their own exemplifies the concept of beneficence in nursing practice. Beneficence refers to the ethical principle of acting in the best interest of the patient, promoting their well-being, and providing care that improves their overall quality of life. By assisting patients with their Activities of Daily Living (ADLs), nurses ensure that their basic needs are met, enhancing their physical and emotional comfort. This act of support goes beyond providing medical treatment and includes helping patients with tasks such as bathing, dressing, grooming, and eating. By enabling patients to maintain their independence and dignity, nurses uphold the principle of beneficence and demonstrate their commitment to holistic patient-centered care.

Question 222:

Correct Answer: A) Habituation

Explanation: In the Neonatal Intensive Care Unit (NICU), it is observed that a newborn named Ethan initially turns his head in response to the sound of a monitor alarm. This behavior indicates a normal auditory response. However, with repeated exposure to the alarm throughout the day, Ethan eventually stops reacting to it. This diminished response is known as habituation. Habituation occurs when an individual becomes less responsive or attentive to a repeated or prolonged stimulus. In Ethan's case, the continuous exposure to the monitor alarm leads to a decrease in his reaction, as his brain becomes accustomed to the sound and no longer perceives it as a significant stimulus.

Question 223:

Correct Answer: C) Elevated blood pressure, accelerated heart rhythm, heart rhythm disorders, shivering, and perspiration.

Explanation: Abrupt discontinuation of beta-blocker medication can lead to various physiological manifestations. Hypertension, increased heart rate, cardiac dysrhythmias, tremors, and sweating are the typical signs that a patient might exhibit in such situations. Hypertension occurs due to the sudden withdrawal of the medication, as beta-blockers help control blood pressure. Increased heart rate is a result of the removal of the medication's inhibitory effect on the sympathetic nervous system, which regulates heart rate. Cardiac dysrhythmias may arise due to the abrupt alteration in the balance between the sympathetic and parasympathetic nervous systems. Tremors and sweating are common manifestations of increased sympathetic activity caused by the abrupt cessation of beta-blockers. It is crucial to monitor patients closely to identify these signs and promptly address any potential complications.

Question 224:

Correct Answer: C) The colon

Explanation: The colon is primarily impacted in the case of Hirschsprung disease. This condition, also known as congenital megacolon, affects the large intestine or colon. In individuals with Hirschsprung disease, certain nerve cells, called ganglion cells, are missing in the lower part of the colon. As a result, the affected segment of the colon is unable to relax and move stool effectively, leading to a blockage. This can cause symptoms such as constipation, abdominal distension, and difficulty passing stool. By understanding that the colon is the main area affected by Hirschsprung disease, healthcare professionals can accurately diagnose and manage this condition to ensure optimal outcomes for patients.

Question 225:

Correct Answer: A) No specific treatment

Explanation: No specific treatment is recommended by the American Academy of Pediatrics (AAP) for managing gastroesophageal reflux in preterm newborns. This recommendation is based on several factors. Firstly, most preterm newborns experience gastroesophageal reflux as a normal physiological process, which resolves on its own as the baby grows. Secondly, the potential risks associated with medications or interventions outweigh the benefits in this population. Premature infants have immature organ systems and are more susceptible to the side effects of medications. Therefore, the AAP emphasizes supportive care measures, such as positioning the baby upright during feeding and burping frequently, to alleviate symptoms of reflux. Monitoring the baby's weight gain and overall health is also recommended to ensure adequate growth and development.

Question 226:

Correct Answer: A) Hypoventilation

Explanation: Respiratory acidosis occurs primarily due to hypoventilation. Hypoventilation refers to an inadequate removal of carbon dioxide (CO_2) from the body through the respiratory system. When ventilation is reduced, the body retains more CO_2, leading to its accumulation in the bloodstream. This excess CO_2 combines with water to form carbonic acid, resulting in a decrease in blood pH and the development of respiratory acidosis. Various factors can contribute to hypoventilation, including respiratory muscle weakness, lung diseases, central nervous system depression, or impaired function of the respiratory control centers. Identifying and addressing the underlying cause of hypoventilation is essential in managing and treating respiratory acidosis.

Question 227:

Correct Answer : C) Mrs. Smith will not be able to breastfeed because of the risk of ingesting galactose in the milk.

Explanation: He will not be able to breastfeed because of the risk of ingesting galactose in the milk. Galactosemia is a rare genetic disorder that affects the body's ability to break down galactose, a sugar found in milk and other dairy products. Babies with galactosemia lack the enzyme needed to convert galactose into glucose, leading to a buildup of galactose in the blood. Breast milk contains lactose, which is broken down into galactose and glucose. Therefore, breastfeeding would expose the baby to galactose, which can have serious health consequences. It is important for Mrs. Smith to understand that in order to ensure the health and well-being of her baby, alternative feeding options such as specialized formula will be necessary.

Question 228:

Correct Answer: B) Café au lait spots

Explanation: Café au lait spots are a type of skin condition that could potentially indicate the presence of neurofibromatosis. These spots are typically characterized by smooth, flat patches on the skin that have a light brown color, resembling the shade of coffee with milk. Neurofibromatosis is a genetic disorder that primarily affects the nervous system, causing tumors to develop on nerve tissue. Café au lait spots are one of the most common early signs of neurofibromatosis and can appear anywhere on the body. The presence of multiple café au lait spots, especially if they are larger in size or increase in number over time, may suggest the need for further evaluation and medical attention to determine if neurofibromatosis is present.

Question 229:

Correct Answer: C) Pneumothorax

Explanation: Pneumothorax is the most likely medical condition indicated in the scenario of a newborn baby, baby Charles, who has been diagnosed with hydrops fetalis and is experiencing respiratory distress along with uneven breathing sounds. Pneumothorax refers to the presence of air in the pleural space, the area between the lungs and the chest wall. This condition can occur due to various reasons, such as trauma during childbirth or a tear in the lung tissue. The presence of air in the pleural space can cause the lung to collapse partially or completely, leading to respiratory distress and abnormal breathing sounds. Prompt recognition and treatment of pneumothorax are crucial to prevent further complications and ensure the baby's respiratory stability.

Question 230:

Correct Answer: A) The mother of the newborn

Explanation: The neonate's mother should be the primary point of contact for updates about the baby's health status and inquiries about care decisions. As the biological mother, she holds the ultimate responsibility and authority for making decisions regarding her child's well-being. While the baby's grandmother may be present and involved, it is crucial to respect the mother's role in caring for her newborn. Directing updates and inquiries to the mother not only acknowledges her primary role in the child's life but also empowers her to be actively involved in decision-making and nurturing the bond with her baby. By prioritizing the mother's involvement, healthcare professionals can support her in developing confidence and taking ownership of her child's health and care.

Question 231:

Correct Answer: A) Formoterol (Perforomist)

Explanation: Formoterol (Perforomist) is not recommended for treating a baby experiencing breathing difficulties. This medication belongs to a class of drugs called long-acting beta2-agonists (LABAs) which are primarily used in managing chronic respiratory conditions in adults. Due to the potential risks associated with using LABAs in infants, such as an increased risk of severe asthma exacerbations and adverse effects on growth, it is not considered a suitable option for treating breathing difficulties in babies. Instead, healthcare professionals typically recommend other medications, such as short-acting beta2-agonists like albuterol, which are safer and more appropriate for infants. It is crucial to consult a medical professional for proper evaluation and guidance in managing breathing difficulties in babies.

Question 232:

Correct Answer: A) Polyhydramnios

Explanation: Polyhydramnios, an excessive accumulation of amniotic fluid, could potentially be a significant ultrasound discovery during pregnancy that may suggest the presence of esophageal atresia. Esophageal atresia is a congenital condition where the esophagus, the tube connecting the mouth to the stomach, does not develop properly. When the esophagus is blocked or disconnected, the fetus may not be able to swallow amniotic fluid, leading to its accumulation in the womb. Therefore, the presence of polyhydramnios is a notable finding that can indicate the possibility of esophageal atresia. It is crucial for medical professionals to identify this condition early on to ensure appropriate management and care for both the mother and the unborn child.

Question 233:

Correct Answer: A) Sunsetting sign

Explanation: Hydrocephalus in newborn babies can present with various symptoms, but one typical and significant sign is known as the "Sunsetting sign." This refers to the downward deviation of the eyes, where the baby's eyes appear to be fixed in a downward gaze. This symptom occurs due to increased pressure within the brain caused by excess cerebrospinal fluid. The Sunsetting sign is an important indicator of hydrocephalus as it suggests an obstruction or blockage in the flow of fluid, leading to the accumulation of fluid in the ventricles of the brain. Identifying this symptom is crucial for prompt diagnosis and intervention, ensuring appropriate management and prevention of potential complications associated with hydrocephalus in newborn babies.

Question 234:

Correct Answer: B) The parent immediately picks up and comforts the crying infant.

Explanation: The parent immediately picking up and comforting the crying infant is a clear indication of a bond or connection being formed. This act demonstrates the parent's ability to recognize and respond to the needs of their child. It signifies a deep level of understanding and empathy, as the parent is able to provide comfort and reassurance in a time of distress. This immediate response also establishes a sense of trust and security between the parent and the infant. Through this action, the parent is showing their unconditional love and commitment to their child's well-being. Overall, the act of picking up and comforting the crying infant is a powerful display of the bond and connection that exists between a parent and their child.

Question 235:

Correct Answer: C) Respiratory alkalosis

Explanation: Respiratory alkalosis is a potential risk that an intubated newborn baby, who is experiencing hyperventilation, may face. This condition occurs when there is an excessive elimination of carbon dioxide from the body, leading to a decrease in the levels of carbon dioxide in the blood. Hyperventilation, which is characterized by rapid and shallow breathing, can cause the newborn's breathing rate to increase beyond what is necessary. As a result, the baby exhales more carbon dioxide than is being produced, leading to a disruption in the acid-base balance of the body. Respiratory alkalosis can have serious consequences for the newborn, including muscle spasms, seizures, and changes in heart rhythm. Therefore, it is crucial to closely monitor and manage the baby's ventilation to prevent the development of respiratory alkalosis.

Question 236:

Correct Answer: B) Maintain an open stoma

Explanation: Maintaining an open stoma is the primary function of stay sutures after a tracheostomy procedure has been performed. These sutures are placed on either side of the tracheostomy incision and serve to hold the stoma edges in position, preventing them from collapsing or closing. By securing the stoma, stay sutures help ensure a patent airway and facilitate easy access for suctioning, cleaning, and changing of tracheostomy tubes. Furthermore, they provide stability during the healing process and minimize the risk of complications such as infection or accidental decannulation. Overall, the presence of stay sutures plays a crucial role in maintaining the functionality and integrity of the tracheostomy stoma.

Question 237:

Correct Answer: B) Inhibits the collapse of alveoli in the neonate.

Explanation: Prevents alveolar collapse: The pulmonary surfactant is vital in a newborn's body as it plays a crucial role in preventing alveolar collapse. By reducing surface tension within the alveoli, the surfactant ensures that the delicate air sacs in the lungs remain open during exhalation. This prevents alveolar collapse and allows for efficient gas exchange, enabling the newborn to breathe properly. Without sufficient surfactant production, a condition known as respiratory distress syndrome (RDS) can occur, especially in premature infants. RDS can lead to alveolar collapse, making it difficult for the newborn to breathe and potentially causing severe respiratory complications. Hence, the presence of pulmonary surfactant is essential for maintaining lung function and facilitating proper breathing in newborns.

Question 238:

Correct Answer: B) Administer a 5-10 cc warm water flush through the G-tube, and if resistance is encountered, attempt aspiration and further flushing.

Explanation: In the Neonatal Intensive Care Unit, if a preterm baby, such as Baby Jake, has a G-tube fitted and the formula is not flowing properly, it is important for the nurse to take immediate action. The nurse should first flush the tube with 5-10 cc warm water to clear any potential blockages. Following this, the nurse should attempt to aspirate and flush the tube if there is resistance. This approach helps to ensure that the formula can flow smoothly through the G-tube, allowing Baby Jake to receive the necessary nutrition. By promptly addressing the issue and taking these steps, the nurse can prevent any complications that may arise from improper feeding and ensure Baby Jake's well-being.

Question 239:

Correct Answer: A) Insert an orogastric tube of 8-French size or larger.

Explanation: Place an 8-French or larger orogastric tube: When a newborn named Lily, who has a feeding tube and is undergoing CPAP treatment, starts to show signs of abdominal bloating, the best course of action is to place an 8-French or larger orogastric tube. This intervention is crucial as it helps to decompress the stomach and relieve the bloating. By inserting the orogastric tube, excess air and fluids can be removed from the stomach, reducing the discomfort and potential complications associated with abdominal distention. Regular monitoring of the abdomen and reassessment of the feeding regimen should also be conducted to ensure Lily's well-being.

Question 240:

Correct Answer: B) Digital vaginal exam

Explanation: Placenta previa is a condition where the placenta partially or completely covers the cervix, which can lead to severe bleeding during pregnancy. In such cases, performing a digital vaginal exam is strictly not recommended. This procedure involves inserting fingers into the vagina to assess the cervix and can potentially disrupt the placenta, causing significant bleeding. To avoid any unnecessary complications, alternative diagnostic methods such as ultrasound or MRI are preferred to evaluate the placental position. It is crucial to prioritize the safety of the mother and the baby, and therefore, healthcare professionals should exercise caution and refrain from performing digital vaginal exams in suspected cases of placenta previa.

Question 241:

Correct Answer: B) Albuterol

Explanation: Albuterol is the preferred treatment option for chronic lung disease or bronchopulmonary dysplasia leading to bronchospasm. Albuterol is a bronchodilator medication that works by relaxing the smooth muscles in the airways, allowing for easier breathing. It is commonly administered through inhalation, providing rapid relief of bronchospasm symptoms such as wheezing, coughing, and shortness of breath. Compared to other bronchodilators, Albuterol has a faster onset of action and a longer duration of effect, making it an effective choice for managing bronchospasm. It is also well-tolerated, with minimal systemic side effects. Overall, Albuterol's efficacy, safety profile, and ease of use make it the preferred treatment option for chronic lung disease or bronchopulmonary dysplasia associated with bronchospasm.

Question 242:

Correct Answer: C)   Hold the neonate upright for 15 to 20 minutes after feeding.

Explanation: Hold the neonate upright for 15 to 20 minutes after feeding. This is the most suitable course of action for a neonate who has been exposed to drugs and often brings up his feedings. Holding the neonate upright after feeding helps to prevent the reflux of gastric contents into the esophagus, reducing the frequency of vomiting. By keeping the neonate in an upright position, gravity helps to keep the stomach contents in place, minimizing the chances of regurgitation. This position also aids in digestion and allows for better absorption of nutrients. Additionally, holding the neonate upright can help alleviate any discomfort caused by reflux. Therefore, adopting this practice is crucial in ensuring the well-being and optimal feeding experience for the neonate.

Question 243:

Correct Answer: B) Oligohydramnios

Explanation: Oligohydramnios, referring to a deficiency of amniotic fluid, is a condition known to elevate the chances of developing pulmonary hypoplasia. During pregnancy, amniotic fluid plays a crucial role in fetal lung development. It helps to promote lung expansion and growth, allowing the lungs to develop to their full potential. However, when oligohydramnios occurs, there is a decreased amount of amniotic fluid surrounding the fetus, which can restrict the normal development of the lungs. This restriction leads to pulmonary hypoplasia, a condition characterized by underdeveloped and smaller-than-normal lungs. Hence, oligohydramnios significantly increases the risk of developing pulmonary hypoplasia in the fetus, highlighting the importance of maintaining adequate amniotic fluid levels during pregnancy.

Question 244:

Correct Answer: B)   It is typical for parents to maintain continuous emotional disconnection from their infant well beyond the point where the infant demonstrates signs of recovery or survival.

Explanation: It is normal for parents to exhibit persistent emotional detachment from their infant for long after the infant begins to show signs of improvement or survival. This statement is not true. Anticipatory grieving is a natural response that individuals may experience when they are facing the impending loss of a loved one. It commonly occurs when a person is aware of a terminal illness or a life-threatening situation. During this time, individuals may go through a range of emotions, such as sadness, anger, and anxiety. However, it is not normal for parents to emotionally detach from their infant, especially after signs of improvement or survival. In fact, parents typically experience heightened emotional attachment and a deep sense of relief when their child shows signs of improvement. It is important to provide emotional support and understanding to parents during this challenging time.

Question 245:

Correct Answer: C) Postpartum blues

Explanation: Postpartum blues, also known as "baby blues," is the probable diagnosis for a mother, such as Mrs. Danielson, who experiences emotional instability, frequent crying, and feelings of worry a few days after giving birth. Postpartum blues is a common condition that affects many new mothers, typically beginning within the first few days after delivery and lasting for up to two weeks. This condition is characterized by mood swings, tearfulness, anxiety, and irritability. It is important to note that postpartum blues is a temporary and self-limiting condition that does not require medical intervention. However, if the symptoms persist or worsen, it is essential to seek further evaluation from a healthcare professional to rule out postpartum depression or other mood disorders.

Question 246:

Correct Answer: A)   "Spina bifida's formation occurs within the initial month of gestation, so the fall she experienced weeks before delivery is unrelated. "

Explanation: Spina bifida develops during the first month of pregnancy and her fall did not cause this. It is important to reassure Mrs. Smith that her baby's condition is not a result of her fall. Spina bifida is a congenital condition that occurs due to incomplete development of the spinal cord and its protective covering. The exact cause of spina bifida is not fully understood, but it is believed to be a combination of genetic and environmental factors. The majority of cases occur spontaneously and are not related to any specific event or action during pregnancy. It is crucial to provide Mrs. Smith with accurate information and alleviate any guilt or blame she may be feeling. Assuring her that her fall did not cause her baby's spina bifida can help alleviate her concerns and focus on providing the best care for her newborn.

Question 247:

Correct Answer: A)   Metabolic alkalosis

Explanation: Metabolic alkalosis can be inferred from the arterial blood gas results of a prematurely born baby girl in the Neonatal Intensive Care Unit, showing a pH of 7.5, HCO3 of 29, and pCO2 of 37. Metabolic alkalosis is characterized by an increase in the pH level and bicarbonate (HCO3) concentration. In this case, the pH value above the normal range indicates alkalosis, while the elevated bicarbonate level supports the diagnosis. The normal pCO2 value suggests that there is no respiratory compensation occurring. Metabolic alkalosis can be caused by various factors, including excessive loss of gastric acid through vomiting or a nasogastric drain, as is the case with this baby girl. Understanding the acid-base imbalance in neonates is crucial for appropriate management and treatment.

Question 248:

Correct Answer: C) Hypoplastic left heart syndrome

Explanation: Hypoplastic left heart syndrome is a heart disorder that is typically associated with symptoms such as feeble peripheral pulses and cold limbs. This condition occurs when the left side of the heart, including the left ventricle, is underdeveloped and unable to function properly. As a result, the heart is unable to pump enough oxygen-rich blood to the body, leading to reduced blood flow to the extremities. The feeble peripheral pulses and cold limbs are indicators of poor circulation, as there is insufficient blood reaching the peripheral tissues. It is crucial to diagnose and treat hypoplastic left heart syndrome promptly, as it is a life-threatening condition that requires immediate medical intervention, including surgical correction.

Question 249:

Correct Answer: B) Movement and touch

Explanation: The progression of proprioception relies on two key factors: movement and touch. Movement plays a crucial role in proprioceptive development as it provides the necessary sensory input for the brain to understand and interpret the position and motion of our body parts. Through various motor activities and exercises, such as walking, running, and performing coordinated movements, our muscles, joints, and ligaments send signals to the brain, allowing it to create a mental map of our body's position in space. Additionally, touch sensations, including pressure, vibration, and texture, provide further feedback to the brain, enhancing proprioceptive awareness. Together, movement and touch form the foundation for the progression of proprioception, enabling us to navigate and interact with our environment effectively.

Question 250:

Correct Answer: A)   Meconium staining

Explanation: Meconium staining is a term used to describe the presence of a green or yellow tinge on a newborn's umbilical cord. This staining occurs when the baby passes meconium, which is the first stool that is typically thick, sticky, and greenish-black in color. In some cases, meconium can be released before birth, leading to its presence on the umbilical cord. This staining may indicate fetal distress during labor or delivery, as it can be a sign that the baby experienced some level of oxygen deprivation. It is important for healthcare professionals to closely monitor the baby's condition and initiate appropriate interventions if meconium staining is observed.

Question 251:

Correct Answer: B) Toxoplasmosis

Explanation: Toxoplasmosis is a parasitic infection that can be caused by the excrement of domestic felines. This disease is caused by the parasite Toxoplasma gondii, which is commonly found in the intestines of cats. The parasite sheds its eggs, called oocysts, in the cat's feces. These oocysts can survive in the environment for long periods and can be ingested by humans through contact with contaminated soil, water, or food. Once inside the human body, the parasites can invade various organs, including the brain, causing a range of symptoms such as flu-like illness, muscle aches, and swollen lymph nodes. Pregnant women and individuals with weakened immune systems are particularly at risk of severe complications. Preventive measures, such as proper hygiene and avoiding contact with cat feces, are crucial in reducing the risk of Toxoplasmosis infection.

Question 252:

Correct Answer: B) "Can you tell me what you understand about your baby's condition? "

Explanation: When parents of a newborn who is showing signs of improvement become increasingly anxious and repeatedly inquire about the possibility of their baby's death, it is important to respond in a supportive and empathetic manner. By asking the question, "Can you tell me what you understand about your baby's condition?" the healthcare professional initiates a conversation that allows the parents to express their concerns and share their understanding of the situation. This response not only acknowledges the parents' anxiety but also opens the door for a comprehensive discussion. By avoiding repetition of the question and starting with this empathetic prompt, the healthcare professional can address the parents' fears and provide accurate and appropriate information, ultimately helping to alleviate their anxiety and build trust in the medical team's expertise.

Question 253:

Correct Answer: C)   Metabolic acidosis

Explanation: Metabolic acidosis is the type of acid-base imbalance that would suggest the presence of volvulus in a newborn baby with malrotation. In this condition, the blood pH decreases due to an excess of acid or a loss of bicarbonate. Volvulus occurs when the intestine twists, leading to compromised blood supply and subsequent tissue damage. This can result in the accumulation of lactic acid and other metabolic byproducts, leading to metabolic acidosis. Recognizing metabolic acidosis in a newborn with malrotation is crucial, as it indicates a potentially life-threatening condition that requires prompt medical intervention. Therefore, close monitoring of acid-base balance and timely intervention are essential to ensure the well-being of the newborn.

Question 254:

Correct Answer: B)   <<0.50

Explanation: <<0.50 is the recommended FiO2 level to be maintained with noninvasive or mechanical ventilation for a preterm newborn in order to avoid oxygen toxicity. Oxygen toxicity refers to the harmful effects of excessive oxygen exposure, which can lead to damage to the lungs and other organs. Preterm newborns are particularly vulnerable to oxygen toxicity due to their underdeveloped lungs and immature antioxidant defense systems. By keeping the FiO2 level below 0.50, healthcare professionals aim to strike a balance between providing adequate oxygenation and minimizing the risk of oxygen toxicity. This level allows for sufficient oxygen delivery to meet the newborn's respiratory needs while reducing the likelihood of oxidative stress and injury. It is crucial to closely monitor the preterm newborn's oxygen saturation levels and adjust the FiO2 accordingly to maintain it within the optimal range. This individualized approach ensures the delivery of adequate oxygen without subjecting the newborn to the detrimental effects of excessive oxygen levels.

Question 255:

Correct Answer: A) At armpit level

Explanation: At armpit level is the ideal position for the uppermost part of the chest clips in an infant's car seat. This advice is given to parents for several reasons. Firstly, placing the chest clips at armpit level ensures that the seat straps are properly secured across the infant's chest, reducing the risk of the child slipping out or being ejected from the seat in the event of a sudden stop or accident. Additionally, positioning the clips at this level ensures that they are not too high on the child's torso, which could potentially cause discomfort or restrict breathing. By following this guidance, parents can help ensure optimal safety and comfort for their infant while traveling in a car seat.

Question 256:

Correct Answer: B) Respiratory acidosis

Explanation: Respiratory acidosis is suggested by the ABG results of Baby Jane. The pH value of 7.24, along with the elevated PaCO2 level of 56 mmHg, indicates an excess of carbon dioxide in the blood. This imbalance is often caused by inadequate ventilation or impaired respiratory function. The HCO3- level of 25 mEq/L falls within the normal range, suggesting that compensation has not yet occurred. The low PaO2 level of 57 mmHg indicates inadequate oxygenation, which can further contribute to the acidotic state. Additionally, the negative base excess of -4 suggests a metabolic component, which is likely compensatory in nature. Overall, these ABG results indicate that Baby Jane is experiencing respiratory acidosis, highlighting the need for further evaluation and appropriate intervention.

Question 257:

Correct Answer: A)   Increase the frequency of breastfeeding

Explanation: Hyperbilirubinemia related to breastfeeding can occur when there is insufficient milk intake by the newborn, leading to elevated bilirubin levels in the blood. To manage this condition, the best course of action is to increase the frequency of breastfeeding. By doing so, the newborn receives a higher volume of milk, which helps to enhance bowel movements and eliminate excess bilirubin from the body. Additionally, frequent breastfeeding stimulates milk production, ensuring an adequate supply for the baby. It is crucial to ensure proper latch and positioning during breastfeeding to maximize milk transfer. This approach is effective in managing hyperbilirubinemia while maintaining the benefits of breastfeeding for the newborn's overall health and development.

Question 258:

Correct Answer: A) Infants of smaller size and premature gestational age

Explanation: Small size and earlier gestational age are significant factors that contribute the most to the increased loss of insensible water. Infants who are born prematurely or have a smaller body size have an underdeveloped skin barrier, which makes them more prone to water loss. The immature skin of premature babies has a higher transepidermal water loss, leading to increased insensible water loss. Additionally, their decreased fat stores and limited ability to regulate body temperature further contribute to higher water loss. Due to these factors, small size and earlier gestational age are key determinants of increased insensible water loss in infants, requiring careful monitoring and management of their hydration status.

Question 259:

Correct Answer: B) Trisomy 13

Explanation: Trisomy 13, also known as Patau syndrome, is a genetic disorder characterized by the presence of an extra copy of chromosome 13. This condition often leads to a wide range of physical abnormalities and developmental issues. The symptoms described, such as polydactyly (extra fingers or toes), closely spaced eyes, micrognathia (small jaw), microcephaly (smaller than normal head size), cleft lip, and a single crease across the palm, are all commonly associated with Trisomy 13. The presence of these distinct features strongly suggests that the newborn baby in question may be affected by Trisomy 13. It is important to consult with a medical professional for a proper diagnosis and to discuss possible treatment options and support for the child and their family.

Question 260:

Correct Answer: C) Hyperoxia test

Explanation: The Hyperoxia test is the most effective method to distinguish between the cardiac and respiratory origins of central cyanosis. This test involves administering a high concentration of supplemental oxygen to the patient and monitoring their response. If the cyanosis resolves quickly, it indicates a respiratory cause, such as hypoventilation or lung disease. On the other hand, if the cyanosis persists despite the administration of oxygen, it suggests a cardiac cause, such as a right-to-left shunt or congenital heart defect. By analyzing the patient's response to the Hyperoxia test, healthcare professionals can accurately differentiate between these two potential origins of central cyanosis.

Question 261:

Correct Answer: B) Magnesium

Explanation: Magnesium has been found to decrease the risk of neurological issues in prematurely born babies. This essential electrolyte plays a crucial role in various physiological processes, including nerve function and development. Premature infants are particularly susceptible to neurological complications due to their immature nervous systems. Magnesium acts as a neuroprotectant by regulating neurotransmitter release, reducing oxidative stress, and preventing excitotoxicity. It also promotes cerebral blood flow, which enhances oxygen and nutrient delivery to the developing brain. By ensuring adequate magnesium levels in premature babies, healthcare providers can help mitigate the risk of neurological issues and support healthy neurodevelopment.

Question 262:

Correct Answer: C) 30 to 40 mL/kg/day

Explanation: The daily rate at which feeding volumes should be increased for most preterm newborns, after starting with minimal enteral feedings, is typically recommended to be around 30 to 40 mL/kg/day. This gradual increase in feeding volumes ensures a safe and effective transition from minimal enteral feedings to full enteral nutrition. By increasing the volumes at this rate, healthcare professionals aim to prevent complications such as feeding intolerance, necrotizing enterocolitis, and excessive weight gain. This approach allows the preterm newborn's gastrointestinal system to adapt and function optimally, promoting digestive health and nutrient absorption. It is essential to closely monitor the infant's tolerance and response to the increased volumes, making adjustments as necessary based on individual needs and medical guidance.

Question 263:

Correct Answer: C) Tachycardia

Explanation: Tachycardia is a potential impact on the heart when muscle relaxants such as pancuronium bromide, vecuronium, or rocuronium are administered to newborns on mechanical ventilation. Tachycardia refers to an increased heart rate, usually above 100 beats per minute. These muscle relaxants act by blocking the neurotransmitter acetylcholine, which leads to the relaxation of skeletal muscles. However, they can also affect the autonomic nervous system, leading to an imbalance in sympathetic and parasympathetic activities. This imbalance can result in an increase in heart rate, causing tachycardia. It is important to closely monitor newborns receiving these medications to ensure their heart rate remains within a normal range and to promptly address any adverse effects to prevent potential complications.

Question 264:

Correct Answer: C) Chorioamnionitis

Explanation: Chorioamnionitis is a medical condition that is typically indicated by symptoms such as a high temperature, an elevated white blood cell count (more than 15,000 per mm3), rapid heart rate in both the pregnant woman and her unborn child, and a discharge from the vagina filled with pus. Chorioamnionitis refers to an infection of the fetal membranes (amnion and chorion) and the amniotic fluid. It is usually caused by bacteria ascending from the vagina and cervix into the uterus. This condition can pose serious risks to both the mother and the baby, including preterm labor, premature rupture of membranes, and intrauterine infection. Prompt diagnosis and treatment with antibiotics are crucial to prevent further complications and ensure the well-being of both the mother and the unborn child.

Question 265:

Correct Answer: B) The neonate requires tube feeding.

Explanation: The neonate needs gavage feedings, as indicated by a score of 3 on the Infant-Driven Feeding Scales (IDFS) - Readiness Score Description. This score signifies that the infant is not yet ready for oral feedings and requires the administration of nutrition through a tube. Gavage feedings involve delivering milk or formula directly into the stomach using a small, flexible tube that is inserted through the nose or mouth. This method ensures that the neonate receives the necessary nutrients while their oral feeding skills continue to develop. It is important to closely monitor the neonate's progress and work with healthcare professionals to gradually transition them to oral feedings when they demonstrate readiness.

Question 266:

Correct Answer: B) The neonate is positioned vertically, bare except for a diaper, on the caregiver's exposed chest.'

Explanation: Kangaroo care is a method of caring for newborn babies that involves skin-to-skin contact between the baby and the caregiver. In this context, the appropriate positioning for a newborn baby is unclothed (diaper is acceptable), placed vertically on the caregiver's bare chest. This positioning is essential for several reasons. Firstly, placing the baby vertically on the caregiver's bare chest allows for maximum skin-to-skin contact, promoting bonding and emotional connection between the caregiver and the baby. Secondly, the unclothed position helps regulate the baby's body temperature, as the caregiver's body provides warmth and stability. Additionally, this positioning allows for ease of breastfeeding, as the baby can easily access the mother's breast. Overall, the positioning of the newborn baby unclothed and vertically on the caregiver's bare chest is crucial for promoting bonding, regulating body temperature, and facilitating breastfeeding during kangaroo care.

Question 267:

Correct Answer: C) This should be given through a central line.

Explanation: This should be given through a central line. Administering dobutamine via an intravenous route requires caution and adherence to specific guidelines. A central line is necessary for this procedure due to the potential risks associated with peripheral administration, such as local tissue damage or phlebitis. Central lines provide direct access to large central veins, allowing for rapid and efficient drug delivery. Additionally, the use of a central line reduces the risk of extravasation, which can occur when the medication leaks into surrounding tissues. By utilizing a central line, the nurse ensures accurate and safe administration of dobutamine, minimizing potential complications and maximizing therapeutic efficacy.

Question 268:

Correct Answer: B) Calcium

Explanation: Calcium is the mineral level that often decreases following the intravenous administration of Lasix. Lasix, also known as furosemide, is a diuretic medication commonly used to treat conditions such as edema and hypertension. It works by increasing urine production and promoting the excretion of excess fluid and electrolytes. One of the electrolytes affected by Lasix is calcium. This medication can lead to increased urinary calcium excretion, resulting in a drop in calcium levels in the body. This decrease in calcium can have various implications, such as the potential for hypocalcemia, which can manifest as muscle cramps, tetany, and cardiac arrhythmias. It is important to monitor calcium levels during Lasix administration and consider appropriate supplementation if necessary.

Question 269:

Correct Answer: C)   Log the blood pressure as a standard measurement and proceed with the newborn's evaluation.

Explanation: Record the blood pressure as a normal reading and continue the assessment of the newborn. In the neonatal intensive care unit (NICU), it is crucial for a nurse to accurately monitor and document the vital signs of newborn babies. A blood pressure reading of 64/40 in baby Jack may appear low, but it is important to consider that blood pressure norms for newborns differ from those of adults. Neonates have lower blood pressure ranges due to their small size and developing cardiovascular system. Therefore, it is essential to interpret the blood pressure reading within the context of the baby's overall condition. The nurse should continue the assessment of baby Jack, including evaluating his heart rate, respiratory rate, oxygen saturation, and perfusion. This comprehensive assessment will provide a more holistic view of the newborn's health status and guide appropriate interventions if necessary.

Question 270:

Correct Answer: C)   Noisy breathing and dyspnea when crying or feeding

Explanation: Noisy breathing and dyspnea when crying or feeding are characteristic symptoms of tracheomalacia in a newborn baby. Tracheomalacia refers to the weakening or floppiness of the cartilage rings in the trachea, leading to the collapse of the airway during breathing. This collapse can cause noisy breathing, also known as stridor, which is a high-pitched sound heard during inhalation. Additionally, when the baby cries or feeds, the increased respiratory effort can further exacerbate the collapse, resulting in dyspnea or difficulty breathing. These symptoms are typically more noticeable during periods of increased activity or agitation. It is essential to recognize and diagnose tracheomalacia promptly to ensure appropriate management and support for the baby's respiratory needs.

Question 271:

Correct Answer: B)   Respiratory distress

Explanation: Respiratory distress is the most frequent negative impact on a newborn due to a Cesarean section. The process of a Cesarean section involves the surgical delivery of the baby through an incision in the mother's abdomen and uterus. Unlike a vaginal birth, where the baby is naturally squeezed through the birth canal, a C-section does not provide the same benefits for the newborn's respiratory system. This can result in the accumulation of fluid in the baby's lungs, making it harder for them to breathe properly after birth. Respiratory distress can manifest as rapid breathing, grunting, flaring of the nostrils, and a bluish tint to the skin. Prompt medical intervention, including administration of oxygen and respiratory support, is crucial to alleviate the negative impact of respiratory distress on the newborn's health.

Question 272:

Correct Answer: A)   Aorta

Explanation: In the case of transposition of the great vessels, the aorta is another potential vessel that could be involved in this condition. The aorta is the main artery that carries oxygen-rich blood from the heart to the rest of the body. In a normal heart, the aorta arises from the left ventricle, while the pulmonary artery arises from the right ventricle. However, in transposition of the great vessels, the aorta and pulmonary artery are switched, resulting in the aorta arising from the right ventricle and the pulmonary artery arising from the left ventricle. This abnormal positioning can lead to significant cardiovascular complications and impair the normal circulation of blood throughout the body.

Question 273:

Correct Answer: C)   Thrombocytopenia

Explanation: Thrombocytopenia is the most frequently observed blood-related symptom in cases of preeclampsia. This condition is characterized by a decrease in platelet count, which can lead to problems with blood clotting. Thrombocytopenia is commonly seen in preeclampsia due to the dysfunction of the endothelium, the inner lining of blood vessels. The damaged endothelium releases factors that cause platelet aggregation and consumption, resulting in thrombocytopenia. This symptom is significant as it increases the risk of bleeding and can lead to complications such as hemorrhage during childbirth. Therefore, monitoring platelet levels is crucial in managing and accessing the severity of preeclampsia.

Question 274:

Correct Answer: B) To enact precise modifications that yield quantifiable enhancements for a patient cohort.

Explanation: The primary objective of quality improvement in a medical setting is to implement specific changes that result in measurable improvements for a group of patients. This entails a systematic approach to identify areas for improvement, develop strategies, and implement interventions to enhance the quality of care provided. By focusing on specific changes, healthcare professionals can target areas that require attention and address them effectively. The ultimate goal is to enhance patient outcomes, safety, and satisfaction through evidence-based practices and continuous evaluation. This approach ensures that healthcare providers are constantly working towards improving the quality of care and delivering the best possible outcomes for their patients.

Question 275:

Correct Answer: C) Congestive heart failure

Explanation: Congestive heart failure is a potential outcome if coarctation of the aorta is not addressed in a timely manner. This condition occurs when the narrowing of the aorta, which is responsible for carrying oxygen-rich blood from the heart to the rest of the body, is left untreated. As a result, the heart has to work harder to pump blood through the narrowed section, leading to increased pressure and strain on the heart muscle. Over time, this excessive workload can weaken the heart and impair its ability to efficiently pump blood, eventually leading to congestive heart failure. It is crucial to address coarctation of the aorta promptly to prevent such complications and ensure optimal heart function.

Question 276:

Correct Answer: A) 150/min

Explanation: At a rate of 150/min, High-frequency ventilation (HFV) administers small tidal volumes. This technique involves delivering a high-frequency airflow to the patient's lungs, allowing for rapid and shallow breaths. By delivering small tidal volumes at a high rate, HFV aims to optimize gas exchange and minimize lung injury. This technique is particularly useful in patients with conditions such as acute respiratory distress syndrome (ARDS) or neonatal respiratory distress syndrome (NRDS), where conventional mechanical ventilation may not be as effective. HFV offers improved oxygenation and ventilation, while reducing the risk of ventilator-induced lung injury. With a rate of 150/min, HFV ensures efficient delivery of small tidal volumes, promoting better respiratory support in critically ill patients.

Question 277:

Correct Answer: A) The infant's reactions and progress

Explanation: The primary concern of the nurse in a scenario where the parents of a newborn are maintaining contact through video calls should be the infant's reactions and progress. The nurse's focus should be on observing the baby's emotional responses, physical development, and overall well-being during these virtual interactions. By closely monitoring the infant's reactions, such as facial expressions, body movements, and vocalizations, the nurse can assess the baby's level of comfort, engagement, and attachment. Additionally, the nurse must ensure that the parents are provided with accurate and detailed information about the baby's progress, growth milestones, and any concerns that may arise. Regular communication and support are vital to foster bonding between the parents and the newborn, despite the physical distance.

Question 278:

Correct Answer: B) 50 to 60 minutes

Explanation: The typical duration of a sleep cycle for a newborn baby is approximately 50 to 60 minutes. During this time, the baby transitions through different stages of sleep, including light sleep, deep sleep, and REM (rapid eye movement) sleep. These cycles are crucial for the baby's development and overall well-being. During light sleep, the baby may stir or wake up easily, while deep sleep is characterized by a more restful state. REM sleep is important for brain development and is associated with dreaming. Understanding the duration of a newborn's sleep cycle is essential for parents to establish healthy sleep patterns and ensure adequate rest for their little ones.

Question 279:

Correct Answer: B) Turner syndrome

Explanation: Turner syndrome is the likely diagnosis for a newborn baby girl presenting with a webbed neck (cystic hygromata), low-set ears, and widely spaced nipples. Turner syndrome is a chromosomal disorder that affects females and occurs due to the complete or partial absence of one of the X chromosomes. This condition can lead to various physical and developmental abnormalities. The characteristic features of Turner syndrome include short stature, heart defects, kidney abnormalities, and infertility. The presence of a webbed neck, low-set ears, and widely spaced nipples are common physical manifestations of Turner syndrome. Early diagnosis and appropriate medical management are crucial to address the associated health concerns and provide appropriate support for affected individuals.

Question 280:

Correct Answer: B) Posttraumatic stress disorder

Explanation: Posttraumatic stress disorder (PTSD) is a condition that can occur as a result of a traumatic event. In this case, Linda's experience of an unplanned Cesarean section at 32 weeks of pregnancy could have been a distressing and traumatic event for her. The symptoms she is displaying, such as nightmares and hypervigilance, are characteristic of PTSD. Nightmares are a common symptom of PTSD, as the traumatic event is often replayed in the person's mind during sleep. Hypervigilance, on the other hand, is a state of heightened alertness and increased sensitivity to potential dangers, which can be a protective response following a traumatic experience. Therefore, Linda's symptoms strongly suggest that she may be experiencing PTSD as a result of her traumatic birth experience.

Question 281:

Correct Answer: B) Tetralogy of Fallot

Explanation: Tetralogy of Fallot is a well-recognized congenital heart abnormality that is known to cause cyanosis. This condition results from a combination of four heart defects, namely, a ventricular septal defect (VSD), pulmonary stenosis, overriding aorta, and right ventricular hypertrophy. The presence of a VSD allows blood to flow from the right ventricle to the left ventricle, leading to mixing of oxygenated and deoxygenated blood. The pulmonary stenosis restricts blood flow to the lungs, resulting in reduced oxygenation. As a result, a significant amount of deoxygenated blood is pumped out into the systemic circulation, causing the characteristic blue discoloration of the skin, lips, and nail beds, known as cyanosis. Therefore, Tetralogy of Fallot is widely recognized as a congenital heart abnormality that causes cyanosis.

Question 282:

Correct Answer: B) 37.5 °C

Explanation: 37.5 °C is the threshold temperature for defining hyperthermia in terms of core body temperature. Hyperthermia refers to an elevated body temperature that exceeds the normal range. The reason why 37.5 °C is considered the threshold is because it represents a significant increase from the normal body temperature of around 36-37 °C. This threshold indicates a deviation from the body's usual thermoregulatory mechanisms, signaling potential physiological stress and an imbalance in heat production and dissipation. It is important to identify hyperthermia promptly as it can lead to various complications, such as dehydration, heat exhaustion, or even heatstroke. Therefore, monitoring body temperature and recognizing the threshold of 37.5 °C is crucial in diagnosing and managing hyperthermia effectively.

Question 283:

Correct Answer: A) >100,000 per mm3

Explanation: During the initial 72 hours of a newborn being treated with extracorporeal membrane oxygenation (ECMO), it is crucial to maintain a platelet count in the blood of >100,000 per mm3. This level is essential to ensure optimal hemostasis and prevent bleeding complications. Platelets play a crucial role in blood clotting, and a count below this threshold can increase the risk of bleeding, which can be life-threatening for newborns undergoing ECMO. Maintaining the platelet count above >100,000 per mm3 helps to support the integrity of the blood vessels, preventing excessive bleeding and ensuring successful ECMO treatment. Regular monitoring of platelet levels during this critical period is necessary to promptly address any abnormalities and maintain the desired platelet count.

Question 284:

Correct Answer: A) Breakdown

Explanation: Breakdown is the third factor that the Neonatal Skin Condition Score takes into consideration, along with dryness and erythema. Breakdown refers to the breakdown of the skin's protective barrier, leading to skin damage and potential injury. This factor assesses the severity of any skin breakdown present, such as erosions, ulcers, or skin tears. It is an essential aspect to consider in evaluating the overall neonatal skin condition as it indicates the extent of skin compromise and the need for appropriate interventions. By including breakdown as a factor, the Neonatal Skin Condition Score provides a comprehensive assessment of the skin status, ensuring that all aspects of skin health are considered for optimal neonatal care.

Question 285:

Correct Answer: B) 30% to 40%

Explanation: After undergoing 24 hours of phototherapy treatment for hyperbilirubinemia, it is expected that Lucy's bilirubin levels will decrease by 30% to 40%. Phototherapy is a common and effective treatment for newborns with high bilirubin levels. It involves exposing the baby's skin to special lights that help break down and eliminate excess bilirubin. The specific percentage of reduction in bilirubin levels can vary depending on various factors such as the initial bilirubin level, the intensity of the phototherapy, and the baby's overall health. However, on average, a decrease of 30% to 40% is considered a typical response to 24 hours of phototherapy. This reduction in bilirubin levels helps prevent the potential complications associated with high bilirubin levels, such as jaundice.

Question 286:

Correct Answer: C)   Streptococcus Group B infection

Explanation: Group B streptococcus (GBS) is the most likely reason for Noah's current state. GBS is a type of bacteria that can be present in the birth canal and can cause serious infections in newborns. In this case, Noah's mother had a fever during labor, which could indicate an infection, possibly caused by GBS. The prolonged labor and premature birth also increase the risk of infection. GBS infection in newborns can lead to respiratory distress, cyanosis, low body temperature, and lethargy, all of which are symptoms Noah is experiencing. It is crucial to diagnose and treat GBS infection promptly to prevent further complications and ensure the well-being of the infant.

Question 287:

Correct Answer: C)   Endotracheal

Explanation: Endotracheal administration is not advised for giving naloxone (Narcan) to newborns. The rationale behind this lies in the fact that endotracheal administration may not effectively deliver the required dose of naloxone to reverse the effects of opioid overdose in newborns. Unlike adults, newborns have smaller airways, making it more challenging to accurately administer the medication via the endotracheal route. Additionally, the absorption and distribution of naloxone may be compromised when administered through the endotracheal tube. Therefore, alternative methods such as intravenous or intramuscular routes are recommended for the administration of naloxone in newborns, ensuring the prompt and effective reversal of opioid-associated respiratory depression.

Question 288:

Correct Answer: C)   Tenderness at the IV site

Explanation: Tenderness at the IV site is an important symptom to be aware of during a blood transfusion in a premature baby like Lily, who is experiencing anemia. This sign may indicate a possible transfusion reaction. When the IV site becomes tender, it suggests that there may be an inflammatory response occurring due to the transfusion. This tenderness can be a result of various factors, such as an incompatible blood type or an immune response triggered by the introduction of foreign blood. Recognizing this symptom is crucial for healthcare professionals as it allows for prompt intervention and appropriate management to prevent further complications. Monitoring the IV site closely and assessing for tenderness is vital in ensuring the safety and well-being of the premature baby during the blood transfusion process.

Question 289:

Correct Answer: A)   a 30-week-old baby in a closed Isolette incubator

Explanation: A 30-week-old baby in a closed Isolette incubator is the least likely to experience insensible water loss. The closed environment of the Isolette incubator provides a controlled and regulated temperature, humidity, and air circulation, which reduces the evaporation of water from the baby's skin and respiratory passages. This minimizes the loss of water through perspiration and respiration. Furthermore, the incubator helps to maintain a stable microenvironment, preventing excessive heat loss that could lead to increased insensible water loss. In contrast, the open-bed warmer (I) and open bassinet (IV) lack the controlled environment necessary to minimize insensible water loss. Additionally, the baby born en route to the hospital (III) may not have immediate access to an environment that can adequately regulate temperature and humidity, making them more susceptible to insensible water loss.

Question 290:

Correct Answer: C)   Hearing loss

Explanation: Hearing loss is a potential risk that newborn baby Liam is exposed to while undergoing treatment for gram-negative sepsis in the Neonatal Intensive Care Unit (NICU). Although the main concern in this scenario is the potential risk of kidney damage due to the relatively high dosage of gentamicin and ampicillin administered to Liam, it is important to be aware of the other potential side effects of these medications. Gentamicin, in particular, is known to have ototoxic effects, meaning it can cause damage to the auditory system. This can lead to varying degrees of hearing loss, ranging from mild to severe. Therefore, it is essential for healthcare professionals to closely monitor Liam's hearing during and after the treatment to ensure early detection and appropriate management of any potential hearing loss.

Question 291:

Correct Answer: A) The neonate develops hypernatremia.

Explanation: The neonate develops hypernatremia as an adaptive response when experiencing hyponatremia and third spacing while receiving intravenous fluids. This adaptive response occurs due to the body's attempt to compensate for the low sodium levels and fluid accumulation in the interstitial spaces. Hypernatremia, an elevated sodium concentration in the blood, helps restore the osmotic balance by drawing water from the interstitial spaces into the bloodstream. This adaptive response aids in maintaining the body's overall fluid balance and preventing further complications associated with hyponatremia and third spacing. Therefore, the neonate's development of hypernatremia serves as a crucial mechanism to counteract the imbalances caused by fluid shifts and low sodium levels.

Question 292:

Correct Answer: B) Inquiring about the parent's preferred learning method

Explanation: Asking how the parent prefers to learn is the initial approach a nurse should take when instructing a parent on how to manage their infant's feeding tube. This approach recognizes the importance of tailoring the teaching method to meet the parent's individual learning style and needs. By asking this question, the nurse can identify if the parent is a visual learner who benefits from demonstrations and visual aids, an auditory learner who learns best through verbal explanations, or a kinesthetic learner who learns by doing. Understanding the parent's preferred learning style allows the nurse to provide instructions in a way that maximizes comprehension and retention, ultimately enhancing the parent's ability to effectively manage their infant's feeding tube.

Question 293:

Correct Answer: A) Caffeine

Explanation: Caffeine is the preferred medication for managing apnea in prematurely born infants. It is a methylxanthine that acts as a central nervous system stimulant. Caffeine stimulates the respiratory centers in the brain, promoting regular breathing patterns and reducing the frequency of apnea episodes in premature infants. Unlike other medications, caffeine has shown consistent effectiveness in improving respiratory drive and reducing the need for mechanical ventilation. Additionally, caffeine has a wider therapeutic window, making it easier to achieve optimal dosage without causing adverse effects. The use of caffeine in managing apnea in premature infants has been supported by numerous studies and is considered safe and well-tolerated. Therefore, caffeine is the preferred option for managing apnea in prematurely born infants.

Question 294:

Correct Answer: C) One parent should to pass on the gene for the disease to manifest

Explanation: One parent needs to pass on the gene for the disease to occur. This is the primary implication when a disease is classified as autosomal dominant. Unlike autosomal recessive diseases where both parents need to pass on the gene for the disease to manifest, autosomal dominant diseases only require one parent to pass on the gene. This means that if an individual inherits the disease-causing gene from one parent, they have a 50% chance of developing the disease. This mode of inheritance often leads to a higher likelihood of the disease being present in subsequent generations, as affected individuals have a 50% chance of passing on the gene to each of their children. It is important to note that the severity and penetrance of autosomal dominant diseases can vary, with some individuals showing more severe symptoms than others.

Question 295:

Correct Answer: B) Babies delivered by Cesareansection

Explanation: Babies delivered by C-section are more prone to developing Transient Tachypnea (TTN) due to a delay in the clearance of lung fluid. During a vaginal delivery, the baby's chest is compressed, helping to expel the excess fluid from the lungs. However, in a C-section, this compression is missing, leading to a slower absorption of lung fluid. As a result, the fluid accumulates in the baby's lungs, causing TTN. It is important to note that TTN is a temporary condition and typically resolves within a few days. Nonetheless, babies delivered by C-section require close monitoring and, if necessary, may need respiratory support to aid in the clearance of lung fluid and improvement of symptoms.

Question 296:

Correct Answer: A) Minimize exposure to external stimuli.

Explanation: Reduce environmental stimuli is a suitable course of action for a neonate who has been exposed to drugs and is experiencing difficulty sleeping. Neonates are highly sensitive to external factors, and excessive stimulation can further disrupt their sleep patterns. By reducing environmental stimuli, such as minimizing noise, dimming lights, and maintaining a calm atmosphere, the neonate's nervous system can be soothed, promoting better sleep. This approach helps create a conducive environment for the neonate to relax and fall asleep more easily. Additionally, reducing environmental stimuli can also help alleviate any potential discomfort or agitation caused by exposure to drugs, allowing the neonate to experience a more restful sleep.

Question 297:

Correct Answer: B) Nifedipine

Explanation: Nifedipine is generally recognized as the tocolytic agent that has the least impact on the heart rate of a fetus. Nifedipine is a calcium channel blocker that primarily acts on smooth muscle in the walls of blood vessels, which helps to relax and dilate them. This mechanism of action allows for the effective inhibition of uterine contractions, thereby delaying preterm labor. Unlike other tocolytics, such as beta-adrenergic agonists or oxytocin receptor antagonists, nifedipine does not significantly affect fetal heart rate. This characteristic of nifedipine makes it a preferred choice among healthcare professionals when considering the safety and well-being of the fetus during tocolytic therapy.

Question 298:

Correct Answer: A) An opening between the pulmonary and aortic arteries

Explanation: A patent ductus arteriosus, in medical terms, refers to an opening between the pulmonary and aortic arteries. This condition occurs when the ductus arteriosus, a blood vessel that connects the pulmonary artery to the aorta during fetal development, fails to close after birth. The persistence of this opening allows blood to flow from the aorta back into the pulmonary artery, causing a shunting of blood. This leads to an increased workload on the heart and can result in various complications, such as congestive heart failure, pulmonary hypertension, and increased risk of infection. Timely diagnosis and treatment of patent ductus arteriosus are crucial to prevent long-term complications and maintain optimal cardiac function.

Question 299:

Correct Answer: A) Aortic Coarctation

Explanation: Coarctation of the aorta is a medical condition that could be suggested by the symptoms described. This condition involves a narrowing or constriction of the aorta, the main artery that carries oxygen-rich blood from the heart to the rest of the body. The mild breathing difficulties and paleness observed in the newborn baby may be indicative of inadequate blood flow to the lower limbs. The sudden rise in pressure in the upper limbs and drop in the lower limbs could be explained by the narrowing of the aorta, causing increased pressure buildup above the constriction and reduced blood supply below it. The difference in oxygen saturation between the right foot and right hand further supports the possibility of coarctation of the aorta.

Question 300:

Correct Answer: A) Sepsis

Explanation: Sepsis is the primary cause of disseminated intravascular coagulopathy (DIC) in newborn babies. DIC is a condition characterized by the abnormal activation of blood clotting throughout the body, leading to the formation of small blood clots in blood vessels. In newborns, sepsis refers to a severe infection that affects their entire body. When the body detects an infection, it triggers a complex immune response, which can lead to the release of substances that activate blood clotting. In sepsis, this response becomes dysregulated, resulting in widespread clot formation and consumption of clotting factors, ultimately leading to DIC. Therefore, sepsis plays a crucial role in the development of DIC in newborn babies.

Question 301:

Correct Answer: A) Pulmonary hypoplasia

Explanation: Pulmonary hypoplasia is a condition that the nurse should be vigilant for when assessing a newborn baby exhibiting characteristics of Potter facies. Pulmonary hypoplasia refers to the underdevelopment or incomplete development of the lungs, which can lead to severe respiratory distress and potentially life-threatening complications. This condition is commonly associated with Potter facies, which includes features such as epicanthal folds, low-set ears, a smooth philtrum, retrognathia, and widely spaced eyes. The presence of these facial characteristics in a newborn baby may indicate an underlying abnormality in lung development, necessitating close monitoring and immediate intervention to prevent respiratory compromise. Early detection and management of pulmonary hypoplasia are crucial in ensuring the baby's well-being and improving their long-term prognosis.

Question 302:

Correct Answer: C) It affects female newborns only.

Explanation: Turner's syndrome predominantly affects females only. This genetic condition is characterized by the absence or abnormalities of one of the two X chromosomes in females. It is estimated to occur in approximately 1 in 2,500 female births. The missing or altered chromosome can lead to various physical and developmental features, such as short stature, infertility, heart defects, and learning disabilities. While newborn boys can also have chromosomal abnormalities, Turner's syndrome is specifically associated with females due to its genetic nature. Early diagnosis and appropriate medical interventions can help manage the associated health concerns and promote a better quality of life for affected individuals.

Question 303:

Correct Answer: A) Subgalealhemorrhage

Explanation: Subgalealhemorrhage is a medical crisis that can potentially result in hypovolemic shock in a newborn. This condition occurs when there is bleeding between the scalp and the skull, leading to a significant loss of blood volume. The subgaleal space is a potential space filled with loose connective tissue and blood vessels, making it prone to bleeding.   In newborns, subgaleal hemorrhage commonly occurs as a result of birth trauma, especially during difficult deliveries or the use of vacuum or forceps. The prolonged or excessive pressure on the baby's head can cause blood vessels to rupture, leading to significant blood loss. Due to the high vascularity of the scalp, the bleeding can be profuse and quickly result in hypovolemic shock. Hypovolemic shock occurs when there is a severe decrease in blood volume, leading to inadequate perfusion of organs and tissues. In newborns, this can be a life-threatening condition, as their limited blood volume makes them more susceptible to rapid and severe consequences of blood loss. Therefore, prompt recognition and management of subgaleal hemorrhage are crucial to prevent hypovolemic shock and its potential complications in newborns.

Question 304:

Correct Answer: C) Brachial plexus injury

Explanation: During a breech birth, if the arm(s) of a fetus, like baby Thomas, becomes entwined around his head, it can potentially lead to a brachial plexus injury. The brachial plexus is a network of nerves that extends from the spinal cord in the neck down to the shoulder, arm, and hand. When the arms of the fetus are wrapped around the head, it can cause excessive stretching or compression of the brachial plexus, resulting in damage to the nerves. This can lead to weakness, loss of sensation, and even paralysis in the affected arm. Immediate medical attention and intervention are necessary to prevent long-term complications and promote optimal recovery for baby Thomas.

Question 305:

Correct Answer: C) 70%

Explanation: 70% is the approximate percentage of total body water in a full-term newborn. This value is crucial to understand the physiological characteristics of newborns. The high percentage of body water in newborns is attributed to their higher water content compared to adults. This is primarily due to their immature kidneys and limited ability to concentrate urine, leading to increased water loss through urine. Additionally, newborns have a higher surface area-to-body weight ratio, which contributes to greater evaporative water loss. Understanding the percentage of body water in newborns is essential in managing their hydration status, especially in cases of dehydration or fluid overload.

Question 306:

Correct Answer: B) Bilateral choanal atresia

Explanation: Bilateral choanal atresia is the medical term used to describe a condition that obstructs a newborn's ability to breathe shortly after birth. This condition is characterized by the complete blockage of the nasal passages due to the absence or abnormal narrowing of the choanae, which are the openings at the back of the nasal cavity. Bilateral choanal atresia is a rare congenital anomaly that can cause significant respiratory distress, especially during the first few weeks of life. Prompt diagnosis and intervention are crucial to ensure the newborn's oxygenation and prevent potential complications. Treatment usually involves surgical correction to create a pathway for normal breathing, allowing the newborn to thrive and develop without respiratory difficulties.

Question 307:

Correct Answer: C) This condition is a result of clogged skin pores and will naturally resolve without intervention.

Explanation: This is due to plugged pores in the skin and it will go away on its own. The small white spots appearing on your baby's nose and chin are a common condition known as milia. Milia occurs when dead skin cells become trapped in the skin's surface and form small, white, pearly bumps. It is a harmless condition that often occurs in newborns and can also affect adults. The nurse should address the first-time mom's concerns by explaining that milia is a normal occurrence and does not require any treatment. Assure her that it is a temporary condition and will resolve spontaneously as the baby's skin adjusts to the environment. Reassuring the mother and providing education about common newborn skin conditions can help alleviate her worries and foster a sense of confidence in caring for her baby.

Question 308:

Correct Answer: C) 3rd day of life

Explanation: On the third day of life, the procedure of gut priming is typically carried out following a baby's birth. This timing is crucial as it allows for the optimal development and functioning of the baby's digestive system. Gut priming involves the introduction of breast milk or formula into the baby's gastrointestinal tract, which kickstarts the production of important digestive enzymes and promotes the growth of beneficial gut bacteria. The third day of life is chosen because it allows for the initial period of transition and adaptation of the baby's digestive system to pass, ensuring that the gut is ready to receive and process nutrients effectively. By starting gut priming on the third day, healthcare professionals aim to support the baby's nutrition and overall health from the earliest stages of life.

Question 309:

Correct Answer: B) Drug concentrations persist above the minimal effective threshold for an extended duration.

Explanation: Drug levels stay above the minimum effective concentration longer in newborn babies compared to adults or older children. This is due to several physiological factors unique to newborns. Firstly, newborns have a smaller volume of distribution for drugs, meaning the drug is more concentrated in their bodies. Additionally, newborns have an immature liver and kidneys, which are responsible for metabolizing and excreting drugs. As a result, drug clearance is slower in newborns, leading to higher drug levels and prolonged exposure to the drug. It is important to consider these differences when administering intravenous drugs to newborns to ensure appropriate dosing and minimize the risk of adverse effects.

Question 310:

Correct Answer: B) Reliability

Explanation: Reliability is the term used to describe a scenario in a research study where the same tool consistently yields measurements over a certain period of time. It refers to the consistency and stability of the measurements obtained using a particular instrument or tool. In other words, reliability indicates the extent to which a measurement tool produces consistent and dependable results. This is crucial in research as it ensures that the data collected is trustworthy and can be replicated. Reliability is essential for drawing accurate conclusions and making valid inferences from research findings. Researchers strive to establish and maintain reliability to enhance the credibility and validity of their studies.

Question 311:

Correct Answer: C) Performing intubation and implanting an orogastric tube for low intermittent suction.

Explanation: Intubating and inserting an orogastric tube to low intermittent suction should be included in the immediate medical response for a newborn baby diagnosed with congenital diaphragmatic hernia experiencing intense breathing difficulties and uneven breathing sounds. Intubation is a procedure where a tube is placed into the baby's airway to help them breathe. It is essential in this case as the baby is experiencing breathing difficulties. The orogastric tube is inserted through the mouth or nose and into the stomach to decompress the gastrointestinal system, reducing the pressure on the diaphragm. This can help alleviate the symptoms of the hernia. Low intermittent suction is applied to the orogastric tube to ensure continuous removal of gastric contents and to prevent any potential complications. This intervention is crucial to provide immediate relief and stabilize the baby's condition. It helps to improve oxygenation, reduce respiratory distress, and prevent further complications that may arise from the hernia.

Question 312:

Correct Answer: B) 60% to 64%

Explanation: The ideal oxygen saturation level for a newborn baby, like little Emma, one minute after birth should be between 60% to 64%. This range ensures an adequate supply of oxygen to the baby's tissues and organs, supporting their healthy transition from the womb to the outside world. At birth, a baby's oxygen saturation level may initially be lower due to the changes occurring in the respiratory and circulatory systems. However, within one minute, it is essential for the saturation level to rise within the specified range. This ensures that the baby's body receives enough oxygen to meet its metabolic needs, promoting proper organ function, and reducing the risk of complications associated with oxygen deprivation.

Question 313:

Correct Answer: B) Sulfonamides

Explanation: Sulfonamides are medications that should not be administered to infants under two months of age due to the risk of developing kernicterus. Kernicterus is a rare but serious condition characterized by the accumulation of bilirubin in the brain, leading to neurological damage. Sulfonamides, such as sulfamethoxazole, can displace bilirubin from its binding proteins, increasing the levels of free bilirubin in the bloodstream. In infants, whose liver function is not fully developed, this can result in excessive bilirubin crossing the blood-brain barrier and causing harm. Therefore, it is crucial to avoid the use of sulfonamides in this age group to prevent the potentially life-threatening complications associated with kernicterus.

Question 314:

Correct Answer: A) Mrs. Smith is experiencing anticipatory grief

Explanation: Anticipatory grief is a psychological response characterized by emotional withdrawal and avoidance of physical contact in individuals facing the imminent loss of a loved one. In the case of Mrs. Smith, her behavior of avoiding contact with her severely sick newborn baby may indicate anticipatory grief. This response is a natural and common reaction to the overwhelming fear and sadness associated with the potential loss of a child. Mrs. Smith's emotional withdrawal may be her way of protecting herself from further emotional pain and preparing for the potential outcome. It is crucial to provide Mrs. Smith with emotional support and guidance during this difficult time, as anticipatory grief can have profound effects on her mental and emotional well-being.

Question 315:

Correct Answer: A) Forceps-/vacuum-assisted delivery

Explanation: Forceps- or vacuum-assisted delivery is the most commonly linked factor to the occurrence of subgaleal hemorrhages. This procedure involves the use of instruments to assist in the delivery of the baby. During forceps or vacuum-assisted delivery, there is an increased risk of trauma to the scalp and blood vessels in the subgaleal space, which can lead to bleeding. The force applied by the instruments can cause damage to the blood vessels, resulting in subgaleal hemorrhages. It is important to note that subgaleal hemorrhages can be serious and potentially life-threatening for the newborn, as they can lead to significant blood loss and complications. Therefore, it is crucial for healthcare professionals to carefully assess and monitor infants who have undergone forceps or vacuum-assisted delivery for signs of subgaleal hemorrhages.

Question 316:

Correct Answer: B) An infant of 34 weeks, bottle-feeding, necessitates a 0.5 lpm O2 supply to keep SpO2 above 90%

Explanation: A 34-week-old infant who is bottle-feeding and requires 0.5lpm O2 to maintain a SpO2 greater than 90% would justify the use of a nasal cannula for oxygen administration. This situation indicates that the baby is experiencing some degree of respiratory distress and requires supplemental oxygen to support adequate oxygenation. A nasal cannula is a suitable option for oxygen delivery in this case as it provides a low flow of oxygen directly to the nasal passage, allowing for comfortable and efficient oxygen delivery. The use of a nasal cannula ensures that the baby receives the required oxygen concentration while still being able to feed and move freely. It is important to monitor the baby's SpO2 levels closely and adjust the oxygen flow rate as needed to maintain optimal oxygenation.

Question 317:

Correct Answer: B) Higher than in term neonates

Explanation: Greater than in term neonates, the absorption of medications through the skin in preterm babies is influenced by several physiological factors. Preterm infants have an underdeveloped outermost layer of the skin, known as the stratum corneum, which acts as a barrier to drug absorption. This thinner barrier allows medications to penetrate more easily into the bloodstream. Additionally, preterm infants have a higher body surface area to weight ratio compared to full-term babies, leading to a larger surface area available for drug absorption. Furthermore, the immaturity of the liver and kidneys in preterm babies results in reduced drug metabolism and clearance, further enhancing drug absorption. Hence, the increased permeability of the skin and reduced drug clearance contributes to a greater absorption of medications through the skin in preterm babies compared to full-term infants.

Question 318:

Correct Answer: B) Potassium

Explanation: Potassium is a crucial mineral for maintaining the acid-base equilibrium in a newborn's nutrition. This essential nutrient plays a vital role in regulating the pH balance within the body. Potassium acts as an electrolyte, helping to control the fluid levels and acid-base balance in the cells. It works in tandem with sodium to facilitate proper nerve and muscle function, including the muscles involved in digestion. Additionally, potassium is involved in the synthesis of proteins and the metabolism of carbohydrates, which are essential for a newborn's growth and development. Thus, ensuring an adequate intake of potassium is essential for maintaining the delicate acid-base balance necessary for a newborn's overall health and well-being.

Question 319:

Correct Answer: A) To detect neonates with critical congenital heart disease

Explanation: To identify infants with severe congenital heart disease, the primary objective of conducting Critical Congenital Heart Disease (CCHD) tests on newborns is to facilitate early detection and intervention. By actively screening newborns for CCHD, healthcare professionals can identify infants who may require immediate medical attention. This allows for timely diagnosis and subsequent treatment, which can significantly improve the health outcomes of affected infants. Early identification of severe congenital heart disease can prevent potential complications and even save lives. Therefore, CCHD tests play a crucial role in ensuring the well-being of newborns and providing them with the necessary medical support from the earliest stages of life.

Question 320:

Correct Answer: A) Metabolic acidosis

Explanation: Metabolic acidosis is the condition typically observed alongside low blood pressure and reduced blood flow in a newborn baby experiencing shock. Metabolic acidosis occurs when the body accumulates an excessive amount of acid or loses too much base, leading to an imbalance in the body's pH levels. In the context of shock, the reduced blood flow and low blood pressure compromise the delivery of oxygen and nutrients to the tissues, resulting in anaerobic metabolism. This anaerobic metabolism leads to the production of lactic acid, which further lowers the pH levels in the body, causing metabolic acidosis. Therefore, in a newborn baby experiencing shock, the presence of metabolic acidosis serves as a critical indicator of compromised blood circulation and organ perfusion.

Question 321:

Correct Answer: C) Volvulus

Explanation: Volvulus is a gastrointestinal condition that could potentially develop as a result of malrotation. In this condition, the intestine twists upon itself, causing a blockage and impairing the blood supply to the affected area. This twisting can occur due to the abnormal positioning of the intestines during fetal development, known as malrotation. Volvulus is a serious condition that requires immediate medical attention as it can lead to bowel perforation, tissue death, and sepsis if left untreated. Common symptoms include severe abdominal pain, vomiting, and distension. Prompt diagnosis and surgical intervention are crucial to relieve the twist, restore blood flow, and prevent further complications associated with volvulus.

Question 322:

Correct Answer: C) Examine the newborn's entire body for peripheral cyanosis and observe for any retractions or indicators of respiratory distress.

Explanation: Assessing the rest of the newborn's body is crucial in determining the initial course of action when a nurse observes a slight bluish discoloration around the mouth. This assessment is aimed at identifying the presence of cyanosis in the extremities or any signs of respiratory distress, such as retractions. By carefully examining the infant's body, healthcare professionals can gather comprehensive information to make an accurate diagnosis and determine the appropriate intervention. This initial course of action ensures a systematic approach in evaluating the newborn's overall condition, enabling timely and effective intervention if necessary. By emphasizing the importance of this assessment, healthcare providers can promptly address any underlying respiratory or circulatory issues, ensuring the well-being of the newborn.

Question 323:

Correct Answer: A) 393 mg

Explanation: 393 mg of ampicillin should be administered for each dose to baby Lily. To calculate this, we need to convert the weight of the baby from pounds and ounces to kilograms. Since 1 pound is equal to 0.4536 kilograms and 1 ounce is equal to 0.02835 kilograms, we can calculate the weight of the baby in kilograms. Baby Lily's weight is 6 pounds and 8 ounces, which is equivalent to 6.5 pounds or 2.94835 kilograms. Next, we multiply the weight of the baby in kilograms by the prescribed dosage of 400 mg/kg/day. This gives us 1177.34 mg/day. Since the medication needs to be divided into three equal parts for every 8 hours, we divide the total daily dosage by 3. This gives us 392.45 mg per dose. Rounding this value to the nearest whole number, we get 393 mg. Therefore, 393 mg of ampicillin should be administered for each dose to baby Lily in the NICU.

Question 324:

Correct Answer: A) Congestive heart failure

Explanation: Congestive heart failure can be a potential outcome if coarctation of the aorta is not addressed in a timely manner. This condition refers to a narrowing of the aorta, which is the main artery that carries oxygenated blood from the heart to the rest of the body. If left untreated, the narrowed aorta can lead to increased pressure in the heart's left ventricle, causing it to work harder to pump blood. Over time, this increased workload can result in the heart becoming weak and unable to effectively pump blood, leading to congestive heart failure. Therefore, it is crucial to address coarctation of the aorta promptly to prevent the development of this serious and potentially life-threatening condition.

Question 325:

Correct Answer: C) Administer epinephrine

Explanation: Administering epinephrine is the appropriate subsequent course of action if a newborn's heart rate remains low at 40, despite receiving positive-pressure ventilation and chest compressions. Epinephrine is a medication that stimulates the heart, leading to an increase in heart rate and blood pressure. It acts by activating alpha and beta adrenergic receptors in the body. In this critical situation, where other resuscitative measures have been attempted without success, administering epinephrine helps to enhance the newborn's cardiac output and systemic perfusion. It is crucial to address the low heart rate promptly, as it may indicate inadequate oxygenation and circulation, potentially leading to organ dysfunction or even death. Administering epinephrine is a life-saving intervention that should be performed by trained medical professionals in a timely manner.

Question 326:

Correct Answer: A) Meconium aspiration syndrome

Explanation: Meconium aspiration syndrome is the most probable diagnosis for the newborn baby exhibiting signs of respiratory distress, such as retracting with each breath and making a low grunting noise due to rapid breathing. Meconium, the baby's first stool, can be passed into the amniotic fluid before birth, especially if the baby is stressed or deprived of oxygen. If the baby inhales this meconium-stained amniotic fluid into their lungs, it can cause airway obstruction and inflammation, leading to respiratory distress. The symptoms of retracting and grunting are characteristic of respiratory distress in newborns, and when accompanied by meconium staining, it strongly suggests meconium aspiration syndrome as the underlying cause. Early recognition and prompt intervention are crucial in managing and treating this condition to prevent further complications.

Question 327:

Correct Answer: B) Enterovirus

Explanation: Enterovirus is the most frequently observed infection in newborns. This viral infection affects the gastrointestinal tract and can lead to various symptoms such as fever, rash, and respiratory distress. Enterovirus is highly contagious and can easily spread from person to person, making newborns particularly vulnerable due to their immature immune systems. Moreover, newborns often acquire the infection during delivery or through contact with infected individuals. The symptoms of enterovirus infection in newborns can range from mild to severe, with complications such as meningitis, encephalitis, and myocarditis being possible. Therefore, it is crucial to closely monitor newborns for signs of enterovirus infection and take necessary precautions to prevent its spread.

Question 328:

Correct Answer: C) Hypoxia refers to the reduced availability of oxygen at the tissue level, whereas hypoxemia denotes a lowered level of oxygen in arterial blood.

Explanation: Hypoxia is a condition characterized by decreased oxygen availability at the tissue level, while hypoxemia refers to a decrease in the oxygen level specifically within arterial blood. Hypoxia can occur due to various factors such as lung diseases, cardiovascular problems, or reduced oxygen-carrying capacity of the blood. It can lead to tissue damage and organ dysfunction if left untreated. On the other hand, hypoxemia is typically caused by inadequate lung function, decreased oxygen intake, or impaired oxygen transport in the blood. It can be measured by assessing arterial blood gases and is commonly associated with respiratory diseases like pneumonia or chronic obstructive pulmonary disease. Understanding the distinction between hypoxia and hypoxemia is crucial for accurate diagnosis and appropriate management of respiratory and circulatory disorders.

Question 329:

Correct Answer: B) Tenderness at the IV site

Explanation: Tenderness at the IV site is an important symptom to consider when providing a blood transfusion to an anemic premature baby. This symptom may indicate a potential transfusion reaction. Transfusion reactions can occur when the recipient's immune system reacts adversely to the transfused blood. Tenderness at the IV site suggests a localized inflammatory response, which could be an early sign of a transfusion reaction. It is crucial to closely monitor the baby's condition during and after the transfusion, as other symptoms of a transfusion reaction may also manifest, such as fever, chills, rash, difficulty breathing, or changes in blood pressure. Early recognition and prompt management of transfusion reactions are vital to ensure the safety and well-being of the baby.

Question 330:

Correct Answer: C) A patient with AB+ blood can receive blood from a donor of any blood type.

Explanation: A patient with AB+ blood can receive blood from a donor of any blood type. This assertion holds true because individuals with AB+ blood type are considered universal recipients. This means that their red blood cells possess both A and B antigens on their surface, as well as the Rh antigen. As a result, they do not have antibodies that will react against any of the A, B, or Rh antigens. Therefore, when AB+ individuals receive blood from donors of any blood type, their immune system does not mount an immune response against the transfused blood cells. This makes AB+ patients highly compatible with all blood types, allowing them to safely receive transfusions from donors with different blood types.

Question 331:

Correct Answer: C) Prostaglandin E1

Explanation: Prostaglandin E1 (PGE1) is the primary course of action for managing a case of transposition of the great arteries. This medication plays a crucial role in maintaining the patency of the ductus arteriosus, a fetal blood vessel that connects the pulmonary artery and the aorta. By administering PGE1, the ductus arteriosus remains open, allowing for the mixing of oxygenated and deoxygenated blood, which is vital for the survival of infants with transposition of the great arteries. This intervention ensures that oxygen-rich blood can reach the systemic circulation, mitigating the consequences of this congenital heart defect. Therefore, Prostaglandin E1 is the recommended initial step in managing cases of transposition of the great arteries.

Question 332:

Correct Answer: A) Inspiratory stridor

Explanation: Inspiratory stridor is a key symptom that suggests a patient, like Michael, is experiencing paralysis of both vocal cords. Inspiratory stridor refers to a high-pitched, harsh sound that occurs during inhalation, indicating an obstruction in the upper airway. When both vocal cords are paralyzed, they fail to open properly during breathing, creating a narrowing or blockage in the airway. This results in the characteristic inspiratory stridor. It is important to note that other symptoms commonly associated with vocal cord paralysis, such as hoarseness, weak voice, and difficulty swallowing, may not be present in all cases. However, inspiratory stridor is a clear indicator that both vocal cords are affected, requiring prompt medical attention and intervention.

Question 333:

Correct Answer: A) Congenital adrenal hyperplasia

Explanation: Congenital adrenal hyperplasia (CAH) is the primary reason for unclear genitalia in a genetically female newborn. CAH is a genetic disorder that affects the adrenal glands, leading to a deficiency in certain enzymes involved in the production of steroid hormones. In females with CAH, there is an excess production of androgens, which are male sex hormones. This excess androgen production can cause varying degrees of masculinization of the external genitalia in female fetuses, resulting in ambiguous or unclear genitalia at birth. Therefore, when a genetically female newborn presents with unclear genitalia, CAH is often considered as the underlying cause due to its impact on the normal development of female genitalia.

Question 334:

Correct Answer: B) Premature delivery

Explanation: Premature delivery is the primary immediate risk for newborns whose mothers have consumed cocaine during their gestation period. Cocaine use during pregnancy can lead to various complications, including early labor and premature birth. This occurs because cocaine can constrict blood vessels, reducing the blood supply to the developing fetus and potentially causing oxygen and nutrient deprivation. The stimulant properties of cocaine can also trigger uterine contractions, leading to premature labor. Premature infants are at a higher risk of experiencing respiratory distress syndrome, developmental delays, and other health issues due to their underdeveloped organs and systems. Therefore, the primary immediate risk for these newborns is indeed premature delivery.

Question 335:

Correct Answer: A) Neonate exhibiting excessive alertness for a duration of 45 to 60 minutes post-birth and possessing dilated pupils.

Explanation: Overly alert neonate for 45 to 60 minutes after birth and dilated pupils are symptoms that would suggest a mild case of birth asphyxia. An overly alert neonate refers to a newborn who appears unusually awake and active within the first hour after delivery. This can be an indication that the baby's brain received sufficient oxygen during the birthing process. Dilated pupils, on the other hand, occur when the baby's autonomic nervous system responds to the stress of birth by widening the pupils. These symptoms, when observed together, can provide valuable insights into the baby's condition and indicate a mild case of birth asphyxia. It is important to note that the presence of these symptoms does not necessarily guarantee a mild case, and a thorough medical evaluation is always recommended.

Question 336:

Correct Answer: A) The abdomen and chest should rise together.

Explanation: The accurate observation to make when evaluating the respiratory condition of a newborn using the Silverman-Anderson index during inhalation is that the abdomen and chest should rise together. This is an important indicator of normal respiratory function in a newborn. When the abdomen and chest rise together during inhalation, it suggests that the baby is utilizing both the diaphragm and intercostal muscles effectively to take in air. This coordinated movement ensures proper oxygenation and ventilation of the lungs. It is a positive sign that the respiratory system is functioning optimally. Therefore, when assessing a newborn's respiratory condition, it is crucial to observe whether the abdomen and chest rise together during inhalation as a measure of normal respiratory effort.

Question 337:

Correct Answer: A) Rocking movement

Explanation: Rocking movement has been observed to significantly reduce the occurrence of apnea in newborn babies. This gentle back-and-forth motion provides a soothing effect on infants, promoting relaxation and a sense of security. The rhythmic movement helps regulate the baby's breathing pattern, preventing episodes of apnea, where breathing temporarily stops. By mimicking the motion experienced in the womb, rocking movement stimulates the vestibular system, which plays a crucial role in regulating respiration. Furthermore, the repetitive motion has a calming effect on the nervous system, reducing stress and promoting better sleep. Overall, incorporating rocking movement into the care routine of newborns can be an effective strategy for minimizing the occurrence of apnea and ensuring their well-being.

Question 338:

Correct Answer: A) Expiratory stridor

Explanation: Expiratory stridor, a potential observation that the neonatal intensive care nurse may make during the examination of newborn baby Lily diagnosed with tracheomalacia, refers to a high-pitched, noisy breathing sound that occurs during exhalation. Tracheomalacia is a condition characterized by the weakening or collapse of the trachea, which can lead to difficulty in breathing. The presence of an expiratory stridor indicates that the airway is narrowed or obstructed during exhalation, causing this distinct sound. It is crucial for the nurse to recognize and document this observation as it can help in assessing the severity of tracheomalacia and guiding appropriate interventions to ensure optimal respiratory support for baby Lily.

Question 339:

Correct Answer: C) 100 mL

Explanation: The minimum fill volume required to operate an automated peritoneal dialysis machine for a neonate suffering from renal failure is 100 mL. This volume is crucial in ensuring that the machine functions optimally and effectively removes waste products and excess fluid from the peritoneal cavity. By using a minimum fill volume of 100 mL, the machine can adequately circulate the dialysis solution throughout the peritoneal cavity, allowing for efficient exchange of solutes and fluid. Additionally, this volume ensures that the dialysis process is safe for the neonate, as it provides an adequate amount of fluid to maintain hemodynamic stability and prevent dehydration. Therefore, a fill volume of 100 mL is essential for successful automated peritoneal dialysis in neonates with renal failure.

Question 340:

Correct Answer: B) The chance of that happening is very low, about 1 out of 100 pregnancies.

Explanation: The chance of a newborn baby with Down syndrome having siblings with the same condition is very low, about 1 out of 100 pregnancies. This means that the likelihood of future children also having Down syndrome is quite small. Down syndrome is caused by the presence of an extra chromosome, specifically chromosome 21, and it typically occurs randomly. Therefore, the parents' concern about the potential risk to their future children can be reassured by informing them that the chances of having another child with Down syndrome are minimal. It is important to provide them with this information to alleviate their worries and allow them to make informed decisions about expanding their family.

Question 341:

Correct Answer: B) Cerebral palsy

Explanation: Cerebral palsy is a chronic condition frequently associated with Periventricular leukomalacia (PVL). PVL refers to the damage or abnormalities in the white matter of the brain, particularly in the periventricular region. This condition primarily affects premature infants, and the damage to the white matter can disrupt the flow of oxygen-rich blood to the brain, leading to injury. Cerebral palsy is a neurological disorder that affects movement, muscle coordination, and posture. It is often caused by brain damage before, during, or shortly after birth, which aligns with the damage caused by PVL. Therefore, due to the shared association with brain injury, cerebral palsy is frequently observed in individuals diagnosed with Periventricular leukomalacia.

Question 342:

Correct Answer: A) Pneumonia

Explanation: Pneumonia is a condition that is more frequently associated with early-onset neonatal sepsis compared to late-onset neonatal sepsis. This is due to several reasons. Firstly, during the early neonatal period, the immune system of newborns is still developing and is not fully equipped to fight off infections. This makes them more susceptible to respiratory infections such as pneumonia. Additionally, early-onset neonatal sepsis is often caused by vertical transmission of bacteria from the mother to the baby during childbirth, and pneumonia-causing bacteria can easily be transmitted through the respiratory tract. Furthermore, the immature lungs of newborns make them more prone to developing pneumonia when exposed to infectious agents. Therefore, it is crucial to recognize the association between pneumonia and early-onset neonatal sepsis in order to promptly diagnose and treat these vulnerable infants.

Question 343:

Correct Answer: C)   Preterm infants

Explanation: Preterm infants are the group most frequently associated with medication errors in the context of neonatal care. This vulnerable population is at a higher risk due to their immature organ systems, which can affect drug absorption, distribution, metabolism, and elimination. Additionally, preterm infants may require unique dosing calculations and adjustments, making medication administration more complex. The use of multiple medications and medical devices in the neonatal intensive care unit further increases the likelihood of errors. Therefore, healthcare professionals must exercise extra caution when prescribing, preparing, and administering medications to preterm infants to prevent adverse events and optimize their care.

Question 344:

Correct Answer: B)   Hearing loss

Explanation: Hearing loss is a potential health risk that newborn babies infected with cytomegalovirus (CMV) may face. CMV is a common virus that can be transmitted to a developing fetus if the mother becomes infected during pregnancy. The virus can cause damage to the auditory system, leading to hearing loss. This can range from mild to severe, and can affect one or both ears. Hearing loss in infants can significantly impact their language and speech development, as well as their overall cognitive and social development. Early detection and intervention are crucial in managing and minimizing the impact of CMV-related hearing loss on a newborn's long-term health and well-being.

Question 345:

Correct Answer: B) Fluid restriction

Explanation: Fluid restriction is the usual course of treatment for a newborn who has experienced birth asphyxia and is showing symptoms of Syndrome of Inappropriate Antidiuretic Hormone Secretion (SIADH). This treatment approach involves limiting the intake of fluids to prevent excessive water retention and dilution of sodium levels in the body. By restricting fluid intake, the aim is to restore the balance of fluids and electrolytes in the newborn's body, which can help alleviate the symptoms associated with SIADH. It is important to closely monitor the newborn's fluid intake and output, as well as their electrolyte levels, to ensure proper management of this condition. Additionally, the healthcare team may also consider other supportive measures to address any underlying causes or complications related to birth asphyxia.

Question 346:

Correct Answer: B) Respiratory support

Explanation: Respiratory support is the primary purpose for which venovenous ECMO is typically utilized. Venovenous ECMO, or extracorporeal membrane oxygenation, is a life-saving technique used in critical care medicine to provide temporary support for patients with severe respiratory failure. By using a machine to bypass the lungs, venovenous ECMO assists in oxygenating the patient's blood and removing carbon dioxide, allowing the lungs to rest and heal. This therapy is particularly beneficial for patients with conditions such as acute respiratory distress syndrome (ARDS), severe pneumonia, or other lung injuries that do not respond to conventional mechanical ventilation. By starting the explanation with "Respiratory support," we emphasize the main purpose of venovenous ECMO without repetition.

Question 347:

Correct Answer: B) Edwards syndrome

Explanation: Edwards syndrome, commonly known as trisomy 18, is a genetic condition characterized by the presence of an extra copy of chromosome 18 in the cells of the body. This additional genetic material disrupts the normal development and functioning of various organs and systems, leading to a wide range of physical and intellectual disabilities. The condition is named after Dr. John H. Edwards, who first described it in 1960. Edwards syndrome occurs in approximately 1 in 5,000 live births and is more commonly observed in females. It is associated with multiple congenital anomalies, including heart defects, kidney abnormalities, clenched fists, and low-set ears. Edwards syndrome is a serious and life-threatening condition, often resulting in a shortened lifespan and significant medical challenges for affected individuals.

Question 348:

Correct Answer: C) T-cells

Explanation: T-cells play a crucial role in a newborn baby's adaptive immune response. These specialized white blood cells are an essential component of the immune system and are responsible for recognizing and targeting specific pathogens. T-cells are involved in the identification of antigens, which are molecules present on the surface of foreign substances. They then initiate a cascade of immune responses, including the production of antibodies by B-cells and the activation of other immune cells. By recognizing and eliminating harmful pathogens, T-cells contribute to the development of the newborn's immune system and help protect against infections and diseases. Therefore, T-cells are a vital element in the adaptive immune response of newborn babies.

Question 349:

Correct Answer: B) Rocking movement

Explanation: Rocking movement has been observed to effectively reduce the occurrence of apnea in newborn babies. This gentle motion, often provided by parents or caregivers, helps to stimulate the vestibular system and promote respiratory stability. The rhythmic swaying motion of rocking has a calming effect on the baby, which can help regulate their breathing patterns and prevent apnea episodes. Rocking movement also aids in soothing the baby, promoting relaxation and better sleep quality. The repetitive motion of rocking mimics the sensations experienced in the womb, providing a sense of familiarity and comfort to the newborn. Overall, the use of rocking movement as a therapeutic intervention has shown promising results in reducing the occurrence of apnea in newborn babies.

Question 350:

Correct Answer: B) A patient with AB+ blood can accept blood from a donor of any blood type.

Explanation: A patient with AB+ blood can receive blood from a donor of any blood type. This statement holds true due to the unique characteristics of AB+ blood. AB+ blood type is considered the universal recipient, meaning that it does not have antibodies against the A, B, or Rh antigens present in other blood types. Therefore, when AB+ blood is transfused into a patient, there is no risk of an immune response or transfusion reaction. This flexibility allows AB+ individuals to receive blood from donors with any blood type, making them advantageous in emergency situations where blood type matching may be challenging or time-consuming. Overall, the compatibility of AB+ blood with all other blood types makes it a valuable resource in blood transfusions.

Question 351:

Correct Answer: C) Ventricular septal defect

Explanation: Ventricular septal defect is the congenital heart condition that is not associated with cyanosis. This condition occurs when there is a hole in the wall (septum) that separates the two lower chambers (ventricles) of the heart. Unlike other congenital heart conditions such as Tetralogy of Fallot or Transposition of the Great Arteries, which can lead to mixing of oxygenated and deoxygenated blood, ventricular septal defect typically allows blood to flow freely between the ventricles without significant mixing. As a result, oxygenated blood can still reach the body's tissues, which prevents the development of cyanosis. However, it is important to note that in some cases, large ventricular septal defects can lead to other complications that may cause cyanosis.

Question 352:

Correct Answer: A) Between 1 week and 3 months

Explanation: Between 1 week and 3 months is the typical time frame in which symptoms of a late-onset group B streptococcal infection start to manifest. Group B streptococcus (GBS) is a type of bacteria that can cause infections in newborns. While early-onset GBS infections usually occur within the first week of life, late-onset infections tend to develop between 1 week and 3 months after birth. It is important to note that the exact timing can vary from case to case. The symptoms of a late-onset GBS infection can include fever, difficulty feeding, irritability, lethargy, and respiratory problems. Prompt medical attention is crucial if any of these symptoms are observed in a newborn, as GBS infections can be serious and potentially life-threatening.

Question 353:

Correct Answer: B) 1 to 3 mL/kg/hr

Explanation: The minimum urinary output of a newborn baby by the third day should be 1 to 3 mL/kg/hr. This range is important as it indicates proper kidney function and hydration status in a newborn. Adequate urine output is crucial as it helps eliminate waste products, maintain fluid balance, and prevent complications such as dehydration and electrolyte imbalances. The measurement of urinary output is commonly used as a clinical indicator of a newborn's well-being. By ensuring a minimum urinary output of 1 to 3 mL/kg/hr, healthcare professionals can monitor the baby's hydration status and intervene promptly if necessary.

Question 354:

Correct Answer: C) Within 10 minutes

Explanation: Within 10 minutes, the impacts of a dopamine infusion would typically dissipate in a child patient in the Neonatal Intensive Care Unit (NICU). Dopamine is a medication commonly used in the NICU to improve blood flow and heart function in critically ill infants. It acts quickly due to its rapid onset of action, making it an effective treatment option in emergency situations. However, it is important to note that the duration of the medication's effects may vary depending on the individual patient's response, the dosage administered, and the specific condition being treated. Close monitoring by healthcare professionals is crucial to ensure optimal dosing and to promptly address any potential adverse effects.

Question 355:

Correct Answer: C) 10 mL/kg

Explanation: 10 mL/kg is the suggested volume for administering normal saline as a volume expander during the resuscitation of a newborn. This volume recommendation is based on extensive research and guidelines provided by medical professionals. Administering 10 mL/kg of normal saline helps to restore and maintain the appropriate fluid balance in newborns, especially in cases where there is hypovolemia or inadequate circulating blood volume. It is important to note that this recommended volume should be carefully calculated based on the newborn's weight, as overdosing can have adverse effects. By administering 10 mL/kg of normal saline, healthcare providers can effectively support the resuscitation process and ensure the newborn receives the necessary fluids for stabilization.

Question 356:

Correct Answer: C) 24 to 36 hours of birth

Explanation: Around 24 to 36 hours of birth, symptoms of neonatal small left colon syndrome typically start to manifest. This condition, characterized by a shortened or underdeveloped left colon in newborns, commonly presents with symptoms such as abdominal distension, failure to pass meconium, and difficulty with bowel movements. The significance of the 24 to 36-hour timeframe lies in the fact that it corresponds to the transitional period after birth when the baby's gastrointestinal system adapts to extrauterine life. During this critical period, the inadequate function of the small left colon becomes noticeable, leading to the emergence of symptoms. Early identification and prompt medical intervention are crucial for managing neonatal small left colon syndrome effectively.

Question 357:

Correct Answer: C) Evaluate for the presence of a fistula.

Explanation: Assess for fistula should be the subsequent course of action if an imperforate anus is identified during the first postnatal examination of a newborn. An imperforate anus is a congenital condition where the opening to the rectum is blocked or absent. It requires immediate medical attention to prevent complications. Assessing for fistula is crucial as it helps determine the presence of an abnormal connection between the rectum and another nearby structure, such as the urinary tract or reproductive organs. This evaluation is important to guide the subsequent management and surgical intervention. Identifying the presence of a fistula allows healthcare professionals to plan the appropriate treatment strategy, which may involve surgical repair to establish a normal anorectal function. Therefore, prompt assessment for fistula is vital in ensuring the best possible outcome for the newborn.

Question 358:

Correct Answer: C) Down syndrome

Explanation: Down syndrome is a genetic disorder that is often associated with the presence of an atrioventricular septal defect (AVSD) or, in milder cases, a ventricular septal defect (VSD), as observed by a Neonatal Intensive Care Unit nurse. Down syndrome, also known as trisomy 21, occurs when there is an extra copy of chromosome 21. This additional genetic material can disrupt the normal development of the heart, leading to structural abnormalities such as AVSD or VSD. These defects affect the septum, which is the wall separating the chambers of the heart. The presence of AVSD or VSD in a newborn, along with other characteristic features, can often indicate the likelihood of Down syndrome.

Question 359:

Correct Answer: C) That the aspirate drains into a drainage bag and the stomach contents be aspirated at least every 30 minutes

Explanation: To prevent the aspiration of saliva in a newborn with an intestinal obstruction and an NG tube, it is crucial that the aspirate drain into a drainage bag and the stomach contents be aspirated at least every 30 minutes. This is essential because when a newborn has an intestinal obstruction, there is a risk of increased saliva production, which can lead to aspiration if not properly managed. By ensuring that the aspirate drains into a drainage bag, any excess saliva can be safely collected and removed, reducing the risk of aspiration. Additionally, regular aspiration of the stomach contents every 30 minutes helps to keep the airway clear and prevents the buildup of secretions that could potentially be aspirated. These measures are vital in maintaining the respiratory health and overall well-being of the newborn named Lily.

Question 360:

Correct Answer: B) Newborn's Transient tachypnea

Explanation: Transient tachypnea of the newborn (TTN) is the primary reason for respiratory distress syndrome in a newborn baby. TTN occurs when a baby's lungs are unable to clear fluid from their lungs quickly after birth. This results in rapid breathing (tachypnea) and difficulty in maintaining oxygen levels. TTN is most common in babies delivered by cesarean section, as they do not undergo the typical squeezing of the chest during a vaginal delivery, which helps expel lung fluid. Additionally, babies born to mothers with diabetes or who experience a prolonged labor may also be at higher risk for TTN. Although TTN is usually self-limiting and resolves within a few days, close monitoring and supportive care are crucial to ensure the baby's respiratory function stabilizes.

Question 361:

Correct Answer: A) Subgaleal hemorrhage

Explanation: Subgaleal hemorrhage is a potential medical crisis that can result in hypovolemic shock in a neW born baby. This condition occurs when there is bleeding between the scalp and the skull beneath the galea aponeurotica, a fibrous layer of tissue. Subgaleal hemorrhage can be caused by trauma during delivery, particularly when the infant's head is subjected to excessive force or prolonged pressure. The bleeding can be significant, leading to a rapid loss of blood volume and subsequent hypovolemic shock. This condition is particularly concerning in newborns because they have limited blood volume, making them more susceptible to the effects of hypovolemia. Immediate medical intervention, such as blood transfusion and fluid resuscitation, is crucial in treating subgaleal hemorrhage and preventing hypovolemic shock.

Question 362:

Correct Answer: C) HELLP syndrome

Explanation: HELLP syndrome is a potentially life-threatening condition that can occur during pregnancy, typically in the third trimester. It is characterized by a combination of symptoms including discomfort in the right upper quadrant, nausea, vomiting, and high blood pressure. These symptoms are indicative of liver dysfunction, which is a key feature of HELLP syndrome. The condition is often associated with preeclampsia, a pregnancy-related complication that involves high blood pressure and damage to organs such as the liver and kidneys. Prompt diagnosis and management of HELLP syndrome are essential to prevent serious complications for both the mother and the baby.

Question 363:

Correct Answer: B) Unconjugated (indirect) bilirubin

Explanation: Unconjugated (indirect) bilirubin is the specific type of bilirubin that typically rises in newborns with hyperbilirubinemia. Bilirubin is a yellow pigment produced from the breakdown of red blood cells. When red blood cells are broken down, bilirubin is released, and it undergoes a process called conjugation in the liver. However, in newborns, the liver may not be fully developed, leading to an accumulation of unconjugated bilirubin in the blood. This elevation in unconjugated bilirubin levels can result in jaundice, a yellowing of the skin and eyes. Monitoring and managing bilirubin levels in newborns is crucial to prevent complications associated with hyperbilirubinemia.

Question 364:

Correct Answer: C) Formoterol (Perforomist)

Explanation: Formoterol (Perforomist) is not recommended for treating an infant, such as baby James, who is experiencing respiratory distress. Formoterol belongs to a class of medications called long-acting beta-agonists (LABAs), which are primarily used to manage chronic obstructive pulmonary disease (COPD) and asthma in adults. However, the safety and efficacy of Formoterol have not been established in infants and young children. Infants have smaller airways and less developed respiratory systems, making them more susceptible to adverse effects from medications like Formoterol. Therefore, it is essential to avoid using this medication in infants and seek alternative treatments that are specifically approved for their age group.

Question 365:

Correct Answer: B) Within 10 minutes

Explanation: Within 10 minutes, the impact of a dopamine infusion should be expected to dissipate in a young patient in the Neonatal Intensive Care Unit. Dopamine is a medication commonly used in the NICU to improve blood flow and increase blood pressure in critically ill infants. It works by stimulating receptors in the blood vessels, which leads to vasoconstriction and an increase in systemic vascular resistance. However, the half-life of dopamine is relatively short, ranging from 2 to 5 minutes. This means that it is rapidly metabolized and eliminated from the body. As a result, the effects of the drug should begin to wear off within a short period of time, typically within 10 minutes. It is important to closely monitor the patient during this time to ensure that their blood pressure and overall condition remain stable.

Question 366:

Correct Answer: B) Vasospasm

Explanation: Vasospasm is a condition characterized by the sudden constriction or narrowing of blood vessels, leading to reduced blood flow to the affected area. In the case of a newborn with an umbilical artery catheter inserted, the presence of blue discoloration in their feet, also known as "catheter toes," suggests the occurrence of vasospasm. This phenomenon can occur as a result of the catheter irritating the arterial wall, triggering a response in the smooth muscle cells of the blood vessels. The constriction of the vessels reduces blood supply to the toes, resulting in the bluish coloration. It is important to monitor and manage vasospasm promptly to prevent further complications and ensure adequate blood flow to the extremities.

Question 367:

Correct Answer: C) Liver failure

Explanation: Liver failure is a significant health risk that newborns suffering from short bowel syndrome and receiving parenteral nutrition are particularly susceptible to. Parenteral nutrition is a method of providing essential nutrients intravenously, bypassing the digestive system. While this approach is crucial for infants with short bowel syndrome who cannot absorb nutrients properly, it can also strain the liver. The liver plays a vital role in metabolizing and processing nutrients, and the high levels of glucose, lipids, and amino acids in parenteral nutrition can overwhelm the liver's capacity. Consequently, this can lead to liver damage and potentially progress to liver failure. Therefore, it is crucial to closely monitor liver function in newborns receiving parenteral nutrition to mitigate the risk of liver failure.

Question 368:

Correct Answer: C) 36 °C to 36.5 °C

Explanation: The optimal skin temperature range for premature babies should be maintained at 36°C to 36.5°C. This specific range is crucial for their well-being due to several reasons. Firstly, maintaining a consistent and appropriate temperature helps in preventing hypothermia, which is a common challenge for premature infants. Secondly, this range ensures that the baby's metabolic rate remains stable, promoting proper growth and development. Additionally, it helps regulate the baby's heart rate, respiratory rate, and oxygen consumption, all of which are vital for their overall health. By keeping the skin temperature within this range, healthcare professionals can provide the necessary warmth without subjecting the baby to overheating, minimizing the risk of complications.

Question 369:

Correct Answer: B) Methicillin

Explanation: Methicillin is typically the preferred method of treatment for staphylococcal infections in newborns due to its effectiveness in targeting the bacteria responsible for the infection. Staphylococcal infections, particularly caused by methicillin-resistant Staphylococcus aureus (MRSA), can be challenging to treat as they are resistant to many commonly used antibiotics. However, Methicillin, a member of the penicillin class of antibiotics, is specifically designed to combat these resistant strains. It works by inhibiting the growth of the bacteria and preventing them from reproducing. Methicillin is often administered intravenously to ensure adequate absorption and distribution throughout the body, allowing it to effectively target the infection. Additionally, its use in newborns is carefully monitored to ensure the appropriate dosage and minimize potential side effects.

Question 370:

Correct Answer: C) Medical negligence

Explanation: Medical negligence refers to a situation where a healthcare professional, in this case, a nurse, fails to provide the standard level of care resulting in harm or unfavorable outcomes for the patient. In the scenario described, if a nurse mistakenly administers an incorrect amount of medicine to a baby in the Neonatal Intensive Care Unit (NICU), leading to adverse consequences, it would be deemed as a case of medical negligence. This term emphasizes the importance of adhering to established protocols, maintaining accurate medication administration, and ensuring the safety and well-being of patients, particularly vulnerable neonates in the NICU. It is imperative for healthcare professionals to exercise utmost caution and precision in their duties to prevent such unfortunate incidents from occurring.

Question 371:

Correct Answer: B) 65 to 75 dB

Explanation: Music therapy for premature babies is an effective intervention that provides numerous benefits for their development and well-being. When utilizing music therapy, it is suggested to maintain a volume level of 65 to 75 dB. This specific range is recommended to ensure that the music is audible and engaging for the baby without causing any discomfort or overstimulation. Research has shown that music played at this volume level can have a soothing effect on premature infants, promoting relaxation, reducing stress levels, and even improving sleep patterns. Moreover, this volume level allows the baby to fully experience the therapeutic benefits of the music without overwhelming their delicate sensory system. Therefore, maintaining a volume level of 65 to 75 dB is crucial in optimizing the effectiveness of music therapy for premature babies.

Question 372:

Correct Answer: B) Human donor milk is provided by a milk bank.

Explanation: Human donor milk is provided by a milk bank. Milk banks are facilities that collect, screen, and process human breast milk from carefully screened and tested donors. These milk banks ensure that the donated milk is safe, pasteurized, and free from any contaminants. The milk is then made available to infants who are unable to receive their mother's milk for various reasons. The accurate statement regarding human donor breast milk is that it is sourced from a milk bank, which acts as an intermediary to ensure the safety and quality of the milk before it is provided to infants in need.

Question 373:

Correct Answer: C) 4 to 7 cmH2O

Explanation: The typical range for maintaining positive end-expiratory pressure (PEEP) in an intubated and ventilated newborn is 4 to 7 cmH2O. This range has been determined based on extensive research and clinical experience. PEEP is an essential component of mechanical ventilation in newborns as it helps to maintain lung recruitment, improve oxygenation, and prevent alveolar collapse during expiration. By applying a positive pressure at the end of expiration, PEEP helps to keep the airways open, increasing functional residual capacity and improving gas exchange. However, it is crucial to individualize PEEP levels based on the specific needs of each newborn, taking into consideration factors such as gestational age, lung compliance, and oxygen requirements. Therefore, the target range of 4 to 7 cmH2O ensures optimal respiratory support while minimizing potential complications associated with excessive or inadequate PEEP levels.

Question 374:

Correct Answer: A) <<0.6 mg/dL (<<10 Î¼mol/L)

Explanation: <<0.6 mg/dL (<<10 μmol/L) is considered the standard range for direct bilirubin levels in a newborn baby. Direct bilirubin is a breakdown product of red blood cells and is processed by the liver. This range signifies the normal and healthy functioning of the liver in the newborn. Maintaining this range is crucial as elevated levels of direct bilirubin can indicate liver dysfunction or other underlying medical conditions. Monitoring direct bilirubin levels helps in the early detection of liver-related issues and allows for timely intervention if necessary. It is important for healthcare professionals to regularly assess direct bilirubin levels in newborns to ensure their overall health and well-being.

Question 375:

Correct Answer: B) 4 hours

Explanation: When it comes to continuous enteral feedings, it is recommended that breast milk or formula be prepared and hung for a duration of 4 hours. This timeframe ensures the safety and quality of the feedings for the patient. Hanging the feedings for longer durations may increase the risk of microbial contamination and subsequent infection. It is crucial to adhere to the recommended duration to minimize the potential for bacterial growth and maintain the nutritional integrity of the breast milk or formula. Regularly replacing the feeding bag and tubing every 4 hours helps to ensure the patient receives a fresh and uncontaminated supply of nutrients.

Question 376:

Correct Answer: B) The neonate has a normal CSF glucose level.

Explanation: The newborn has a normal CSF glucose level. Glucose is the primary source of energy for the brain, and its level in the CSF is tightly regulated. A normal CSF glucose level typically ranges between 50-80 mg/dL in neonates. Lily's CSF glucose level of 100 mg/dL falls within this range, indicating that her brain is receiving an adequate supply of glucose. Abnormal CSF glucose levels can be indicative of various conditions such as meningitis or metabolic disorders. However, since Lily's CSF glucose level is within the normal range, it suggests that her brain function is not compromised by any underlying medical conditions.

Question 377:

Correct Answer: B) Obstruction in the chest tube

Explanation: Obstruction is the likely cause if no visible fluctuation is observed in the chest tube or the bottle of a newborn baby, named Lily, who has a chest tube inserted due to pneumothorax. This lack of fluctuation indicates that there is a blockage or obstruction in the chest tube, preventing the normal movement of air and fluid. It could occur due to a kink or twist in the tube, blood clots, or tissue debris. Obstruction in the chest tube can impede the drainage of air or fluid from the pleural space, potentially leading to complications such as lung collapse or infection. Timely identification and resolution of the obstruction are crucial to ensure proper functioning of the chest tube and promote Lily's recovery.

Question 378:

Correct Answer: A) Weight >2,000 g

Explanation: Weight >2,000 g is one of the crucial requirements for a newborn to be eligible for extracorporeal membrane oxygenation (ECMO). ECMO is a life-saving intervention that provides cardiac and respiratory support to critically ill infants. Infants who require ECMO are usually suffering from severe respiratory or cardiac failure, and their condition is often life-threatening. The weight criterion helps ensure that the newborn's organs and systems are sufficiently developed to withstand the stress of the ECMO procedure. Infants weighing less than 2,000 g may have underdeveloped organs, making them more vulnerable to the potential risks and complications associated with ECMO. Therefore, meeting the weight requirement is essential to ensure the newborn's chances of a successful ECMO treatment.

Question 379:

Correct Answer: C)   Tummy to tummy with the mother reclining

Explanation: Tummy to tummy with the mother reclining is the most effective breastfeeding position for a newborn with a small jaw and feeding difficulties but no breathing issues. This position allows for optimal positioning and alignment of the baby's mouth and jaw, ensuring a proper latch and effective milk transfer. The reclining position of the mother helps to support the baby's head and neck, reducing strain on their jaw muscles. Additionally, the close proximity between the mother and baby in this position promotes bonding and skin-to-skin contact, which can further enhance breastfeeding success. By starting with "Tummy to tummy with the mother reclining" and elaborating on its benefits, we can provide a detailed rationale without repetitive phrasing.

Question 380:

Correct Answer: B)   Colostomy

Explanation: Colostomy is typically the first surgical procedure performed on newborns, such as baby Jane, who are diagnosed with persistent cloaca. This procedure involves creating an opening in the abdomen, known as a stoma, through which the colon is brought to the surface. By diverting the fecal matter away from the affected area, colostomy allows for proper elimination and prevents complications such as infection and bowel obstruction. It provides a temporary solution, allowing the baby to grow and develop before additional surgeries can be performed to reconstruct the affected organs. Colostomy plays a crucial role in managing persistent cloaca and ensuring the overall health and well-being of the newborn.

Question 381:

Correct Answer: C)   Infant formula or breast milk

Explanation: In the initial months after birth, a newborn is capable of digesting proteins found in formula or human milk. These proteins are specifically designed to be easily digested and absorbed by the delicate digestive system of a newborn. Formula and human milk contain proteins that are broken down into smaller, more manageable molecules, such as amino acids and peptides, which can be readily absorbed by the baby's intestines. These proteins provide essential nutrients and contribute to the growth and development of the newborn. Although there are other sources of proteins available, such as solid foods, the primary and most suitable sources for a newborn's digestion during the initial months are formula or human milk.

Question 382:

Correct Answer: A)   Administer a pacifier for the infant to suck during the tube feedings

Explanation: Offering a pacifier to a premature baby during tube feedings can be a beneficial activity to facilitate the transition from tube to oral feedings. The act of sucking on a pacifier provides essential oral stimulation, which helps strengthen the baby's sucking reflex and improves coordination between sucking, swallowing, and breathing. By introducing a pacifier during tube feedings, the baby learns to associate sucking with the feeling of satiety, promoting a positive oral experience. This activity also aids in the development of the baby's oral muscles, jaw, and tongue, essential for successful oral feedings. Furthermore, the pacifier provides comfort and soothes the baby, making the feeding process more enjoyable. Introducing a pacifier during tube feedings can be an effective strategy to encourage a premature baby's transition to oral feedings.

Question 383:

Correct Answer: A)   Ductus arteriosus

Explanation: Ductus arteriosus plays a crucial role in the circulation of blood to the lungs in cases of pulmonary atresia. This condition, characterized by the absence or closure of the pulmonary valve, prevents blood from flowing directly into the pulmonary artery. However, the ductus arteriosus serves as a temporary conduit, allowing blood to bypass the non-functional pulmonary valve and reach the lungs. This vessel connects the pulmonary artery to the aorta, enabling oxygenated blood from the left side of the heart to be shunted directly to the lungs. By maintaining this essential connection, the ductus arteriosus ensures that the developing fetus receives adequate oxygenation before birth.

Question 384:

Correct Answer: C)   Incorrect location of a central venous catheter tip

Explanation: Incorrect location of a central venous catheter tip can be a frequent reason for a cardiac tamponade occurring in a newborn. This occurs when the catheter tip is inadvertently placed within the heart or its surrounding structures, leading to the accumulation of blood or fluids around the heart. This can result in compression of the heart chambers, impairing their ability to fill and pump blood effectively. The incorrect placement of the catheter tip can occur due to various factors, such as improper technique during insertion or inadequate monitoring during placement. Prompt recognition and immediate intervention are crucial to prevent further complications and ensure the newborn's hemodynamic stability.

Question 385:

Correct Answer: A) <<1,250 g

Explanation: 1,250 g is the preterm birth weight that is commonly associated with the highest insensible water loss (IWL). Insensible water loss refers to the amount of water lost through evaporation from the skin and respiratory tract, which is a crucial factor to consider in preterm infants. These infants have a higher IWL due to their immature skin barrier and increased respiratory rate. The weight of 1,250 g is significant because it represents a threshold where infants are more susceptible to fluid loss. Understanding this association is important in clinical practice as it helps healthcare professionals determine appropriate fluid management strategies and prevent complications associated with dehydration in preterm infants weighing less than 1,250 g.

Question 386:

Correct Answer: A) 0.6 mL

Explanation: 0.6 mL of medication should be administered to a newborn if they are prescribed a dose of 0.9 mg and the available concentration of the drug is 1.5 mg per 1 mL. To calculate the required volume, we can use a simple proportion. Since the concentration is 1.5 mg per 1 mL, we can set up the equation: 1.5 mg/1 mL = 0.9 mg/x mL. Cross-multiplying, we get 1.5x = 0.9, and solving for x, we find that x = 0.6 mL. Therefore, to administer the prescribed dose of 0.9 mg, the newborn should be given 0.6 mL of the medication.

Question 387:

Correct Answer: A) 10 mL/kg

Explanation: The appropriate volume of packed red blood cells to administer in a single transfusion for baby Michael, who has been diagnosed with anemia and is showing symptoms of hypoxemia, would be 10 mL/kg. This volume is determined based on the weight of the newborn, with the recommended dosage being 10 mL for every kilogram of body weight. By administering the packed red blood cells in this calculated dosage, the aim is to replenish the oxygen-carrying capacity of the blood and correct the anemia. It is crucial to ensure that the transfusion is carried out accurately and with close monitoring of the baby's vital signs to avoid any complications and to provide effective treatment for this condition.

Question 388:

Correct Answer: B) Bleeding

Explanation: Bleeding is the most commonly observed issue associated with the use of ECMO (Extra Corporeal Membrane Oxygenation). This occurs due to several factors, including the use of anticoagulation medications to prevent clotting within the ECMO circuit. These medications can cause excessive bleeding in some patients. Additionally, the insertion of cannulas into major blood vessels can lead to vessel injury, resulting in bleeding. Furthermore, the ECMO circuit itself can cause damage to blood components, leading to bleeding complications. Managing and preventing bleeding in ECMO patients requires close monitoring of coagulation parameters, adjusting anticoagulation therapy, and employing strategies to minimize trauma during cannula insertion and circuit handling. Ultimately, recognizing and addressing bleeding complications promptly is crucial to ensure the safety and success of ECMO therapy.

Question 389:

Correct Answer: A) Prolactin

Explanation: Prolactin is the hormone that is released in higher amounts when a mother's nipples are stimulated. This hormone plays a crucial role in lactation and is responsible for the production of breast milk. When a baby suckles at the mother's breast, it stimulates nerve endings in the nipple, which then sends signals to the brain. In response to these signals, the brain releases prolactin from the pituitary gland. Prolactin then stimulates the milk-producing cells in the breast, leading to an increased production of breast milk. This hormone is essential for the successful initiation and maintenance of breastfeeding. Therefore, the release of prolactin in higher amounts when a mother's nipples are stimulated is vital for ensuring an adequate milk supply for her baby.

Question 390:

Correct Answer: C) Fetal alcohol syndrome

Explanation: Fetal alcohol syndrome, indicated by certain head and facial characteristics such as small eyes, an unusually thin upper lip, lack of a philtrum, and a smaller than average head size, is a condition that arises due to maternal alcohol consumption during pregnancy. This syndrome occurs when alcohol passes from the mother's bloodstream through the placenta and affects the developing fetus. The characteristic facial features observed in newborns with fetal alcohol syndrome are distinct indicators of this condition. It is crucial to identify and diagnose fetal alcohol syndrome early on, as it can lead to various developmental and cognitive impairments in the affected child. Understanding the connection between these specific facial features and the condition helps healthcare professionals provide appropriate care and support for affected infants like Lily.

Question 391:

Correct Answer: B) Infants being able to feed sooner

Explanation: Infants being able to feed sooner is a significant potential outcome when a cycled lighting system, which is bright in the daytime and dim at night, is implemented in the Neonatal Intensive Care Unit (NICU). This lighting system helps mimic the natural circadian rhythm, which plays a crucial role in regulating feeding patterns in newborns. By exposing infants to bright light during the day and dim light at night, their internal body clock is better aligned, promoting increased wakefulness during the day and improved sleep at night. As a result, infants may exhibit improved feeding behaviors, such as increased appetite, more effective sucking, and better digestion. This, in turn, can lead to earlier establishment of oral feeding, faster weight gain, and overall better nutritional outcomes for the infants in the NICU.

Question 392:

Correct Answer: C) Improper positioning of the central venous catheter tip

Explanation: Incorrect location of a central venous catheter tip is a frequent reason for cardiac tamponade in newborn babies. This occurs when the catheter, which is placed in a large vein to deliver fluids or medications, is inserted too far and ends up in the heart. As a result, the catheter can damage the heart's structures, leading to bleeding and the accumulation of blood or fluid in the pericardial sac, causing cardiac tamponade. This condition is dangerous as it puts pressure on the heart, impairing its ability to pump blood effectively. Prompt recognition and intervention are essential to prevent further complications and ensure the baby's well-being.

Question 393:

Correct Answer: C) 8CM

Explanation: 8CM is the estimated distance from the lips to the midpoint between the glottis and carina for an endotracheal tube in a newborn baby weighing 2 kg, as per the 7-8-9-10 rule. This rule provides a guideline for determining the appropriate endotracheal tube insertion depth based on the infant's weight. The rule suggests that for a newborn weighing 2 kg, the tube should be inserted to a depth of 8 cm. This depth is crucial to ensure proper placement and function of the endotracheal tube, allowing for effective ventilation and oxygenation of the baby's lungs. It is important to adhere to these guidelines to minimize the risk of complications and optimize the infant's respiratory support.

Question 394:

Correct Answer: B) Elevated secretion of catecholamines

Explanation: Increased release of catecholamines is crucial for maintaining glucose balance in a newborn's body after birth. Catecholamines, such as epinephrine and norepinephrine, are hormones released by the adrenal glands in response to stress or low blood glucose levels. These hormones stimulate glycogenolysis, which is the breakdown of stored glycogen into glucose. In newborns, glycogen stores are essential as the primary source of glucose until they establish regular feeding patterns. The increased release of catecholamines helps mobilize glycogen stores and ensures a steady supply of glucose to meet the energy demands of the newborn. This mechanism is vital for maintaining glucose homeostasis and preventing hypoglycemia, a condition that can have adverse effects on the newborn's neurological development.

Question 395:

Correct Answer: A) Immediately prior to administering the standard scheduled dosage.

Explanation: Just before giving a regular scheduled dose, a blood sample should be taken from a baby in the Neonatal Intensive Care Unit who is being treated with carbamazepine (Tegretol) for seizures in order to check the drug level. This timing is crucial as it allows the healthcare professionals to monitor the concentration of the drug in the baby's system. By measuring the drug level just before administering the next dose, the medical team can ensure that the dosage is appropriate and within the therapeutic range. Regular monitoring of the drug level helps to optimize the treatment and minimize the risk of adverse effects or inadequate seizure control. Therefore, obtaining a blood sample right before the scheduled dose is essential for effective management of the baby's seizures.

Question 396:

Correct Answer: A) Washing with water and allowing it to air dry

Explanation: Cleansing a newborn's umbilical cord with water and allowing it to dry is the recommended method for its care. This approach is essential to prevent infection and promote healing. By gently cleaning the cord stump with water, any debris or bacteria can be removed, reducing the risk of infection. After cleansing, it is crucial to ensure the cord is completely dry, as moisture can create an environment for bacterial growth. This method is simple, safe, and effective in promoting healing and preventing complications. By following this approach, parents can provide the best care for their newborn's umbilical cord and ensure a smooth transition to a healthy belly button.

Question 397:

Correct Answer: A) Chronic hypoxia

Explanation: Chronic hypoxia is frequently the underlying cause of polycythemia associated with hyperviscosity. When an individual experiences prolonged oxygen deprivation, their body responds by producing more red blood cells in an attempt to compensate for the lack of oxygen. This excessive production of red blood cells leads to an increased viscosity of the blood, resulting in a condition known as polycythemia. Chronic hypoxia can arise from various factors, such as lung diseases, high altitude living, or certain heart conditions. It is crucial to address the underlying cause of chronic hypoxia to prevent further complications and manage the symptoms associated with polycythemia and hyperviscosity.

Question 398:

Correct Answer: C) Sepsis

Explanation: Sepsis is the most probable condition that can arise as a result of early onset group B strep infection in a newborn. Sepsis refers to a severe systemic infection that can occur when bacteria, such as group B strep, enter the bloodstream and spread throughout the body. In the case of early onset group B strep infection, the bacteria can be transmitted from the mother to the baby during childbirth. Once the bacteria enter the baby's body, they can quickly multiply and cause an overwhelming infection. This can lead to sepsis, where the body's immune response becomes dysregulated and can result in organ dysfunction and failure. Sepsis is a medical emergency that requires prompt diagnosis and treatment to prevent serious complications and potentially save the newborn's life.

Question 399:

Correct Answer: C) 4.6 to 8 mg/dL (1.5 to 2.6 mmol/L)

Explanation: The standard range for serum phosphorus levels in a newborn baby is 4.6 to 8 mg/dL (1.5 to 2.6 mmol/L). This range is considered normal and healthy for newborns. Serum phosphorus levels play a crucial role in various physiological processes, such as bone development, energy metabolism, and acid-base balance. It is essential for the proper functioning of the nervous system, muscles, and kidneys. Maintaining the appropriate phosphorus levels is particularly important during the early stages of life when babies are experiencing rapid growth and development. Deviations from this standard range can indicate underlying health conditions and may require medical intervention. Regular monitoring of serum phosphorus levels in newborns ensures optimal health and well-being.

Question 400:

Correct Answer: B) 2 mg/kg/day beginning at 2 months

Explanation: 2 mg/kg/day beginning at 2 months is the suggested dosage of additional iron for a preterm neonate with low birth weight. This dosage is recommended to address the increased iron requirements of preterm infants, as they are at a higher risk of iron deficiency anemia due to their rapid growth and limited iron stores at birth. Administering iron supplementation at this dosage helps in preventing and treating iron deficiency, which can have adverse effects on the baby's neurodevelopment and overall growth. It is important to note that this dosage is specific to preterm neonates with low birth weight, and individualized dosing based on the infant's weight and response to treatment should be determined by a healthcare professional.

Question 401:

Correct Answer: A) Renal abnormalities

Explanation: Renal abnormalities are the primary reason for high blood pressure in a prematurely born infant. The kidneys play a crucial role in regulating blood pressure by filtering waste products and excess fluids from the bloodstream. In premature infants, the kidneys may not have fully developed, leading to structural and functional abnormalities. These renal abnormalities can disrupt the normal process of fluid and electrolyte balance, resulting in increased blood pressure. Additionally, immature renal blood vessels and impaired autoregulation further contribute to elevated blood pressure in premature infants. It is important to closely monitor and manage blood pressure in these infants to prevent complications and ensure optimal growth and development.

Question 402:

Correct Answer: B) Vitamin K

Explanation: Vitamin K is the specific vitamin needed for the liver to produce procoagulant factors and regulatory proteins. This essential vitamin plays a crucial role in blood clotting or coagulation. The liver synthesizes various proteins that are involved in the coagulation cascade, including prothrombin, factors VII, IX, and X. These proteins rely on vitamin K to undergo a process called carboxylation, which enables them to function effectively in blood clotting. Without sufficient vitamin K, the liver's ability to produce these vital proteins would be compromised, leading to impaired blood clotting and an increased risk of bleeding. Therefore, vitamin K is essential for the proper functioning of the liver in maintaining hemostasis.

Question 403:

Correct Answer: C) Thiazide diuretics (hydrochlorothiazide)

Explanation: Thiazide diuretics, such as hydrochlorothiazide, have the potential to elevate the levels of calcium in the serum. These diuretics work by inhibiting the reabsorption of sodium and chloride in the distal convoluted tubules of the kidneys, leading to increased excretion of fluid and electrolytes, including calcium. Due to their mechanism of action, thiazide diuretics reduce calcium excretion, resulting in higher levels of calcium in the bloodstream. This effect is particularly beneficial for individuals with conditions such as hypercalciuria or kidney stones, where reducing calcium excretion can help prevent stone formation. However, it is important to monitor serum calcium levels regularly when using thiazide diuretics, as excessively high calcium levels can have adverse effects on various body systems.

Question 404:

Correct Answer: B) The trach tube can be reused after it has been cleaned properly.

Explanation: The trach tube can be reused after it has been cleaned properly. This crucial information is important for caregivers to understand when a nurse is providing instructions on home-based tracheostomy care. Proper cleaning and disinfection of the trach tube is essential to prevent the risk of infection and ensure the patient's safety. Caregivers need to comprehend the correct technique and frequency of cleaning, as well as the appropriate cleaning solutions to use. They should also be aware of the importance of maintaining a sterile environment during the cleaning process. By understanding these instructions, caregivers can effectively manage and maintain the tracheostomy care at home, promoting the patient's well-being and reducing the risk of complications.

Question 405:

Correct Answer: B) Hypocalcemia

Explanation: Hypocalcemia is a medical condition characterized by low levels of calcium in the blood. In newborn babies, signs of jitteriness in the limbs could be indicative of hypocalcemia. Calcium plays a crucial role in muscle contraction and nerve function, and when its levels are low, it can lead to increased neuromuscular excitability, resulting in jitteriness or tremors in the limbs. This condition is particularly concerning in newborns as calcium is essential for proper development and functioning of the nervous and muscular systems. Therefore, identifying hypocalcemia as the medical implication in a newborn baby showing signs of jitteriness is crucial for prompt diagnosis and appropriate management to prevent any potential complications.

Question 406:

Correct Answer: C) Sepsis

Explanation: Sepsis is a life-threatening condition that occurs when the body's response to an infection damages its own tissues and organs. In the case of an early onset group B strep infection in a newborn baby, sepsis can be the probable cause. Group B streptococcus (GBS) is a bacterium commonly found in the vaginal or rectal area of pregnant women. During childbirth, the baby can be exposed to GBS, leading to an infection. If the infection spreads rapidly and affects the bloodstream, it can result in sepsis. Newborns are particularly vulnerable to sepsis as their immune systems are not fully developed. Therefore, it is crucial to identify and treat GBS infections promptly to prevent the onset of sepsis in newborn babies.

Question 407:

Correct Answer: B) Primary cytomegalovirus infection at birth

Explanation: Congenital cytomegalovirus infection is the primary reason for infants experiencing hearing impairment. This viral infection, caused by the cytomegalovirus (CMV), can be transmitted from the mother to the fetus during pregnancy. CMV is a common virus that often goes undetected in adults, but it can have severe consequences for a developing fetus. The virus can affect the inner ear and auditory nerve, leading to hearing loss in infants. It is estimated that about 1 in every 200 infants is born with congenital CMV infection, making it a significant cause of hearing impairment in this population. Early detection and intervention are crucial in managing and minimizing the impact of hearing loss in infants with congenital cytomegalovirus infection.

Question 408:

Correct Answer: A)   Reducing the amount of feed administered

Explanation: Decreasing the feeding volume may be a suitable intervention for a newborn baby who has a feeding tube and is experiencing vomiting, but shows no signs of any physical issues. Vomiting in a newborn can occur due to various reasons, such as overfeeding or intolerance to the formula being used. By reducing the amount of milk or formula being administered, the baby's digestive system can have more time to process and tolerate the feedings. This intervention aims to prevent overwhelming the baby's digestive capacity, giving it an opportunity to adjust gradually. It is important to closely monitor the baby's response to the decreased volume and consult with a healthcare professional to ensure optimal nutrition and health.

Question 409:

Correct Answer: B)   Nonmaleficence

Explanation: Nonmaleficence is the ethical principle being applied in the situation where parents decide to opt for palliative care only for their newborn with severely compromised health. Nonmaleficence, also known as the principle of "do no harm," guides healthcare professionals to prioritize the avoidance of harm or suffering to the patient. In this scenario, the doctor has informed the parents that continued treatment may only extend the baby's discomfort without offering any significant improvement to their health. By choosing palliative care, the parents are prioritizing the relief of their baby's suffering and ensuring a peaceful and comfortable end-of-life experience. This decision aligns with the principle of nonmaleficence as it aims to prevent further harm or unnecessary discomfort to the newborn.

Question 410:

Correct Answer: A)   Hypertension

Explanation: Hypertension, or high blood pressure, is a clear indication that a baby might be experiencing an excess of fluids in their system. This condition occurs when there is an abnormal increase in the pressure within the blood vessels. In infants, hypertension can present itself through various signs, such as irritability, excessive sweating, rapid weight gain, and difficulty breathing. Additionally, the fontanelle (soft spot on the baby's head) may appear bulging or tense. These symptoms may also be accompanied by a decrease in urine output and swelling of the extremities. Hypertension in babies should never be ignored, as it can lead to serious complications if left untreated. It is crucial for parents to seek immediate medical attention if they suspect their baby is experiencing an excess of fluids in their system, as early diagnosis and treatment are essential for the well-being of the infant.

Question 411:

Correct Answer: A)   Infant formula or breast milk

Explanation: Formula or human milk are the primary sources of nutrition for newborns in the initial months after birth. These sources contain proteins that are easily digestible by the newborn's developing digestive system. The proteins found in formula or human milk are specifically designed to meet the nutritional needs of infants, providing them with essential amino acids necessary for growth and development. These proteins are generally in a more easily digestible form, such as whey proteins, which are quickly broken down and absorbed by the newborn's immature digestive system. Therefore, formula or human milk is the ideal choice for providing the necessary proteins for a newborn's growth and development in the first few months of life.

Question 412:

Correct Answer: B) Hunger

Explanation: Hunger is the primary indicator of the newborn's behavior such as nodding their head, clenching their hands, and smacking their lips. These actions signify that the baby is seeking nourishment. As a nurse, it is important to inform novice parents about these cues to help them understand their baby's needs. By recognizing these hunger cues, parents can respond promptly by offering breastfeeding or formula feeding to ensure their baby's adequate nutrition. It is crucial for parents to be aware that these behaviors are the newborn's way of communicating their hunger, and by responding appropriately, parents can establish a healthy feeding routine and promote their baby's growth and development.

Question 413:

Correct Answer: A)   The neonate has only cleft lip and palate

Explanation: The neonate has only cleft lip and palate. In this scenario, both environmental and genetic influences play an equal role in the occurrence of cleft lip and palate. Cleft lip and palate are a complex condition that can be caused by a combination of genetic factors and environmental exposures during pregnancy. Genetic factors can contribute to the development of cleft lip and palate by affecting the formation and fusion of the facial structures during early embryonic development. On the other hand, environmental factors such as maternal smoking, alcohol consumption, certain medications, and nutritional deficiencies can also increase the risk of cleft lip and palate. Therefore, the presence of only cleft lip and palate in a neonate suggests that both genetic and environmental influences have contributed equally to the occurrence of this condition.

Question 414:

Correct Answer: B)   Brow bulge with vertical furrows

Explanation: Brow bulge with vertical furrows is a significant facial expression that signifies physical discomfort and suffering in a newborn baby. This expression is characterized by the wrinkling of the forehead, specifically in the area between the eyebrows. It is often accompanied by a pained or distressed expression on the baby's face. The brow bulge with vertical furrows is commonly observed when the baby is experiencing discomfort, such as when they are in pain, hungry, or have a discomforting sensation like gas or a wet diaper. Recognizing this facial expression is crucial for caregivers and medical professionals as it helps to identify and address the baby's needs promptly, ensuring their comfort and well-being.

Question 415:

Correct Answer: A)   Total bilirubin encompasses both direct and indirect bilirubin, whereas direct bilirubin refers to the unconjugated portion that typically transits from the liver to the small intestine.

Explanation: Total bilirubin is the amount of direct and indirect bilirubin, while direct bilirubin is the unbound amount of bilirubin that normally passes from the liver to the small intestine. The distinction between these two assessments lies in the different forms of bilirubin they measure. Total bilirubin includes both direct and indirect bilirubin, which are formed during the breakdown of red blood cells. Direct bilirubin, on the other hand, specifically measures the unbound bilirubin that is processed by the liver and excreted into the small intestine. Understanding the levels of total bilirubin and direct bilirubin is crucial in assessing liver function and diagnosing various liver disorders such as jaundice, hepatitis, and cirrhosis. Elevated levels of total bilirubin indicate a potential issue with the liver's ability to process bilirubin, whereas elevated levels of direct bilirubin may suggest a blockage or dysfunction in the bile ducts. By differentiating between total and direct bilirubin, healthcare professionals can gain valuable insights into the underlying causes of liver dysfunction and tailor appropriate treatment plans accordingly.

Question 416:

Correct Answer: C)   Ethan is experiencing severe polyuria

Explanation: Severe polyuria is the preliminary understanding of Ethan's situation. Polyuria refers to excessive urine production, and in this case, Ethan has produced 100 mL of urine in the last four hours. Considering his weight of 6 lbs. (approximately 2.73 kg), this amount of urine output is significantly higher than what is expected for a baby of his size. Severe polyuria can indicate an underlying kidney disease, which aligns with Ethan's diagnosis. It is crucial for the neonatal intensive care nurse to further investigate the cause of this excessive urine production and monitor Ethan's condition closely to ensure appropriate management and treatment.

Question 417:

Correct Answer: B)   Biliary atresia

Explanation: Biliary atresia is the likely medical indication for a newborn if the test results reveal a high level of conjugated (direct) bilirubin in their blood serum. Biliary atresia is a rare but serious condition that affects the bile ducts outside and inside the liver. It occurs when the bile ducts are blocked or absent, leading to the accumulation of bilirubin in the blood. This condition can result in jaundice, pale stools, dark urine, and an enlarged liver. Prompt diagnosis and treatment are crucial to prevent further liver damage and complications. Biliary atresia often requires surgical intervention, such as the Kasai procedure or liver transplantation, to restore proper bile flow.

Question 418:

Correct Answer: B)   Differential cyanosis

Explanation: Differential cyanosis is the most likely type of cyanosis being displayed in this case. This condition is characterized by a mismatch in oxygenation between the upper and lower parts of the body, resulting in a pink coloration in the upper body and a blue coloration in the legs and toes. The presence of a noticeable murmur further supports this diagnosis. Differential cyanosis can occur when there is a cardiac defect that causes a right-to-left shunt of blood, leading to deoxygenated blood bypassing the lungs and entering the systemic circulation. This can result in inadequate oxygenation of the lower extremities, hence the blue coloration. The breathing rate of 55 breaths per minute and heart rate of 120 beats per minute may be indicative of the baby's compensatory response to the decreased oxygen levels.

Question 419:

Correct Answer: B) Increased PaCO2

Explanation: In the event of metabolic alkalosis and a rise in HCO3-, the compensatory process is an increase in PaCO2 to maintain acid-base balance. Increased PaCO2 (partial pressure of carbon dioxide) helps to counterbalance the elevated bicarbonate levels by stimulating the respiratory system to increase ventilation. This leads to an increase in the elimination of carbon dioxide through the lungs, resulting in a decrease in blood pH and a compensatory effect for the metabolic alkalosis. By emphasizing the answer and avoiding repetition of the question, it is clear that the compensatory process for metabolic alkalosis and elevated HCO3- levels is an increased PaCO2 through respiratory adjustments.